Thieme

The Practice of Ultrasound

A Step-by-Step Guide to Abdominal Scanning

Berthold Block, M. D.
Private Practice
Braunschweig
Germany

900 Illustrations
36 Tables

Georg Thieme Verlag
Stuttgart · New York

Library of Congress Cataloging-in-Publication Data is available from the publisher.

This book is an authorized translation of the 2nd German edition published and copyrighted 2003 by Georg Thieme Verlag, Stuttgart, Germany. Title of the German edition: Der Sono-Trainer: Schritt-für-Schritt-Anleitungen für die Oberbauchsonographie.

Translator: Terry C. Telger, Fort Worth, TX, USA
Illustrators: Viorel Constantinescu, Bucharest and Jörg Decker, Stuttgart

© 2004 Georg Thieme Verlag
Rüdigerstraße 14, 70469 Stuttgart, Germany
http://www.thieme.de
Thieme New York, 333 Seventh Avenue, New York, NY 10001 USA
http://www.thieme.com

Cover design: Martina Berge, Erbach-Ernsbach
Typesetting by Ziegler + Müller, Kirchentellinsfurt
Printed in Germany by Grammlich, Pliezhausen

ISBN 3-13-138361-5 (GTV)
ISBN 1-58890-280-3 (TNY)

1 2 3 4 5

Preface

Health care professionals who want to practice abdominal ultrasound are often faced with two obstacles:

1. Colleagues rarely have the time or inclination to train new operators.
2. Standard textbooks of ultrasonography give little attention to the typical problems of beginners.

This book is designed as a self-study guide for those who want to learn ultrasound scanning one step at a time. Several underlying principles are followed:

1. The chapters are arranged so that the book can be used during an ultrasound examination. It should be placed next to the examination couch. In this way the examiner can learn all about ultrasound anatomy in small, manageable steps. By referring to the concise text and matching illustrations, the user can quickly reproduce the technique that is being described. The scan may be performed on a patient, on a colleague, or even on the user himself.
2. Every sectional ultrasound image is two-dimensional. The image is "brought to life" by moving the transducer over the body surface to create a three-dimensional impression of what is being scanned. For this reason, the ultrasound visualization of anatomic structures is illustrated by a sequence of images, rather than by a single image as in most other books.
3. Three-dimensional artwork. Instead of showing a flat coronal view, for example, the anatomical drawings provide a "sliced" view of structures that shows just how the structures are cut by the sector-shaped beam. As source materials for these perspective views, the author used ultrasound image sequences, computed tomographic scans, and anatomical sections, depending on the requirements of the situation.

The author hopes that this introduction will provide a complete and easy-to-use guide to the practice of upper abdominal ultrasound. I wish the reader enjoyable reading and successful scanning.

Braunschweig, Spring 2004   Berthold Block

Acknowledgments

I express my thanks to the following colleagues, who either contributed images that I did not have in my own files or supplied me with images of better quality.

Dr. med. Stefan Hänel
Herzogin Elisabeth Heim Hospital
Hochstrasse 11
38102 Braunschweig

PD Dr. med. Meinolf Karthaus
Evangelisches Johannes Hospital
Medical Clinic
Schildescher Strasse 99
33611 Bielefeld

Dr. med. Bernd Krakamp
Medical Clinic I
Cologne Municipal Clinics
Merheim Hospital
Ostmerheiner Strasse 200
51109 Cologne

Dr. med. Ingo Krenz
Schlankreye Dialysis Center
Schlankreye 38
20144 Hamburg

Dr. med. Ralf Kuhlmann
Braunschweig Medical Center
Celler Strasse 38
38114 Braunschweig

Prof. Dr. med. Bernd Limberg
Medical Clinic
Municipal Hospital
Alter Weg 80
38302 Wolfenbüttel

Dr. med. Johannes Linder
Medical Clinic I
Braunschweig Medical Center
Salzdahlumer Strasse 90
38126 Braunschweig

Dr. med. Hilmar Milbradt
Neustadt am Rübenberge
District Hospital
Lindenstrasse 75
31535 Neustadt am Rübenberge

I extend special thanks to PD Dr. med. Hartmut Schmidt of the University Medical Center Charité in Berlin. I also thank Mr. Viorel Constantinescu for turning my rough sketches into precise sectional diagrams.

The great majority of ultrasound images were obtained with a Siemens scanner. The author is grateful to the Siemens Corporation for generously providing the scanner on loan.

I thank the staff at Thieme Medical Publishers for their constant and courteous help and support, especially Dr. Antje Schönpflug and Mrs. Claudia Güner for their valuable advice during the production phase.

I express very special thanks to Dr. Markus Becker of Thieme Medical Publishers, who encouraged me throughout the creation of this book and supported me in every way.

Berthold Block

Table of Contents

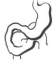

11 Adrenal Glands 230

12 Bladder, Prostate, and Uterus 236

13 The Systematic Ultrasound Examination 241

1 General

How to Use This Book

This book is a self-study guide, designed to enable you to begin scanning a live subject right away, without any prior theoretical knowledge of ultrasonography. Different readers will have different degrees of experience with ultrasound. Therefore the book is structured so that you can access the material at your own level of knowledge and experience. Because the book is practice-oriented, less emphasis is placed on physical and technical details, which are basically limited to the following three questions:

LEARNING GOALS

➤ Who do you examine first when learning ultrasound?
➤ How do you adjust the ultrasound machine?
➤ What can you do with the transducer?

After addressing these questions, we will cover the practical aspects of performing an upper abdominal ultrasound examination according to a standardized routine. The protocol for examining the major abdominal organs — the liver, gallbladder, pancreas, kidneys, spleen, vena cava, and aorta — proceeds from the simple to the more complex:

First, you locate the organ of interest and demonstrate it in its entirety. Second, you define the organ details. Third, you evaluate the relations of the organ to surrounding structures.

In theory, then, there are two basic strategies for scanning the upper abdomen:

➤ Organ-oriented: an organ or structure is identified, scrutinized, and evaluated in relation to surrounding structures.
➤ Level-oriented: the abdominal organs are examined as a whole, proceeding in steps. First, all of the abdominal organs are successively located and surveyed. Next the organ details are defined, and finally the interrelationships of all the organs are evaluated.

In practice, you will generally apply a combination of both strategies. But in all cases you will learn to follow a structured, step-by-step protocol that is the essence of systematic upper abdominal ultrasound.

Smaller organs and structures of the upper abdomen will be covered in a less formalized way: the stomach, duodenum, porta hepatis, and adrenal glands.

KEY POINTS

Locate and survey the organ.

Define the details of the organ.

Define its relations to neighboring structures.

Examination Technique and Equipment

Who do you examine first when learning to scan?

You should select a young, slender, fasting subject and examine him or her in the morning if at all possible. If you meet these criteria yourself, you should know that self-examination can be mastered with very little practice. You just have to reorient your thinking compared with examining another person, and this can be done relatively quickly.

How do you adjust the ultrasound machine?

The ultrasound system consists of the ultrasound machine itself, the transducer (probe), and the monitor (screen). Each of these elements affects the quality of the examination.

Ultrasound machine

As a beginner, you should not try to learn all the fine points of "knobology" right away. You should, however, be familiar with all of the functions shown in Fig. 1.1.

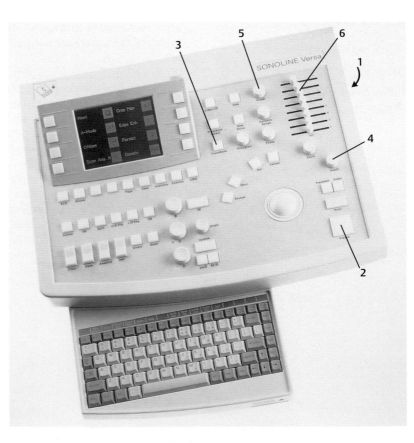

Fig. 1.1
Control panel of an ultrasound machine.
1 On/off switch
2 Freeze button
3 Transducer selector switch
4 Penetration depth
5 Power output
6 Time-gain compensation (TGC)

On switch. Turns the machine on and off.

Freeze button. If the machine was used earlier, the previous operator may have activated the freeze button, locking out all the function switches. In this case you must turn off the freeze switch before using the machine.

Transducer selector switch. More than one transducer may be available for use. You can choose the desired transducer with a selector switch. To begin with, select the 3.5 MHz curved array. Further details on this type of transducer are given below.

Penetration depth. You turn a knob to set the penetration depth of the ultrasound scan. This has the effect of widening or narrowing the image field. Start with the control set to 12 cm. Most of the images in this book were obtained at this setting.

Power output, overall gain, and time-gain compensation. Recall for a moment the way that diagnostic ultrasound works. Ultrasound waves are transmitted, partially reflected by tissues, and received. The intensity of both the transmitted waves and the received signals can and should be adjusted and optimized. The power transmitted by the system, called the power output, affects the brightness of the image. A low power output produces a dark image, while a high power output yields a bright image. The overall gain also affects image brightness. A dark image at a low power setting can be brightened by increasing the gain, and a bright image can be darkened by lowering the gain. Both functions should be carefully balanced to obtain a quality image. A good general rule is to set the power output to the lowest possible level. On the other hand, setting the gain too high to compensate for a low power setting will produce a "noisy" image. Through practice, you will learn how to achieve a proper balance.

Every ultrasound machine has two gain controls. The overall gain control is used to amplify the received echoes over the entire depth of the image field. The time-gain compensation (TGC) amplifies echoes according to their depth to achieve uniform image brightness.

TIP

Set the power output to an intermediate setting, and move all the TGC slide switches to the center. Adjust the overall gain to obtain good mid-field brightness. Now adjust the slide switches to produce uniform brightness in the near and far fields. When this is done correctly, the slide switches will usually form an approximate diagonal line.

Transducers

Three different transducers are important for routine scanning: the sector transducer, linear transducer, and curved array (Fig. 1.2).

Sector transducer (Fig. 1.2a). In a sector transducer, the ultrasound beam is moved through a fan-shaped sector either mechanically (by rotary movement of the transducer elements) or electronically (by sequential firing of the elements). The ultrasound image is narrow at close range and widens out with distance from the transducer face.
> Advantages: small footprint, ability to scan through a small acoustic window, clear definition of structures at greater depths.
> Disadvantage: poor resolution of structures near the transducer.

Linear transducer (Fig. 1.2b). In a linear transducer, multiple parallel elements are arranged in a straight line, producing a rectangular image field.
> Advantage: good resolution of structures near the transducer.
> Disadvantages: large footprint, cannot scan through a narrow acoustic window close to the transducer.

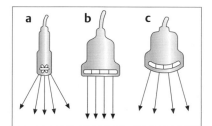

Fig. 1.2
Principal transducer designs.
a Sector transducer
b Linear transducer
c Curved array

Curved array (Fig. 1.**2c**). In a curved array, the piezoelectric elements are lined up as in a linear transducer, but on a convex surface. This produces a fan-shaped image similar to that of a sector transducer but considerably wider in the near field.
➤ Advantage: compromise between a sector and linear transducer.
➤ Disadvantage: line density decreases with depth, as in a sector transducer.

Frequency. Besides the shape of the transducer and the arrangement of the elements, image quality is determined by the frequency of the emitted sound. Frequencies in the range of 2.5 to 7.5 MHz are generally used for diagnostic ultrasound. High frequencies provide less penetration depth with higher resolution, while low frequencies give deeper penetration with lower resolution. Transducers with an operating frequency of 3.5 MHz are commonly used for upper abdominal scanning. Most of the images in this book were obtained with a 3.5 MHz curved array.

Adjusting the monitor

You can adjust the monitor's brightness and contrast. Adjust the brightness level so that you can distinguish the background brightness of the monitor image from the structures surrounding the image. Then adjust the contrast to a level at which you can distinguish all shades of gray in the gray bars.

What can you do with the transducer? _____

You use the transducer to obtain a two-dimensional sectional image of the body that is displayed on the monitor. Structures located closer to the transducer are displayed at the top of the screen, and structures farther away are displayed at the bottom. All other localizing information — right/left, cranial/caudal, lateral/medial, and posterior/anterior — depends on how the transducer is positioned.

Transducer position

To aid in understanding the transducer and how it is positioned, we will first reduce the infinite number of possible scan planes through the body to three cardinal planes of section: transverse, longitudinal, and coronal.

Transverse section. The transducer is placed to scan a cross section of the body. Structures located on the right side of the body may be displayed on the left or right side of the screen, depending on how the transducer is rotated. You should always position the transducer so that the right side of the body is displayed on the left side of the screen. You will then be viewing the section from below upward, as in a CT scan (Fig. 1.**3**).

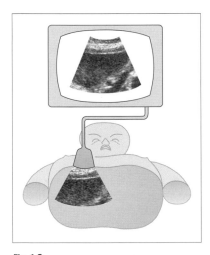

Fig. 1.3
Plane of section of a transverse scan.

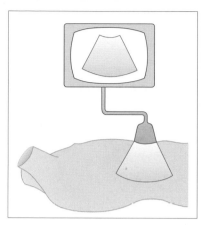

Fig. 1.**4**
Plane of section of a longitudinal scan.

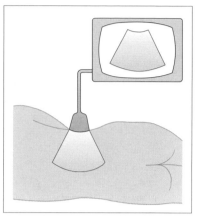

Fig. 1.**5**
Plane of section of a coronal scan from the right side.

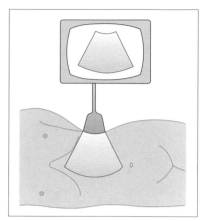

Fig. 1.**6**
Plane of section of a coronal scan from the left side.

Longitudinal section. The transducer is placed parallel to the long axis of the body. Cranial or caudal body structures may be displayed on the left side of the screen, depending on how the transducer is rotated. Always place the transducer so that cranial structures appear on the left side of the screen, i.e., you are looking into the body from right to left (Fig. 1.**4**).

KEY POINT

The three cardinal planes of section through the body are: transverse, longitudinal, and coronal.

Coronal section. The transducer is placed on the side of the body to scan a frontal (coronal) section. As in a longitudinal scan, position the transducer so that cranial body structures are displayed on the left side of the screen and caudal structures on the right. Anterior/posterior orientation depends on whether you are scanning from the patient's right or left side. With a coronal scan from the right side, you are viewing the body from the back (Fig. 1.**5**). When you scan from the left side, you are viewing the body from the front (Fig. 1.**6**).

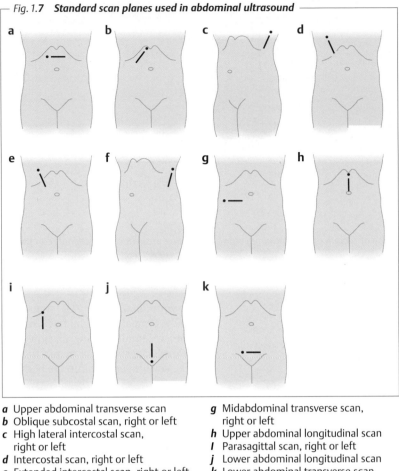

Fig. 1.7 **Standard scan planes used in abdominal ultrasound**

a Upper abdominal transverse scan
b Oblique subcostal scan, right or left
c High lateral intercostal scan, right or left
d Intercostal scan, right or left
e Extended intercostal scan, right or left
f Flank scan, right or left
g Midabdominal transverse scan, right or left
h Upper abdominal longitudinal scan
i Parasagittal scan, right or left
j Lower abdominal longitudinal scan
k Lower abdominal transverse scan

Routine scan planes. Now you know the three standard planes for routine scanning: transverse, longitudinal, and coronal. These planes can be combined in an infinite variety of ways, of course, but a limited number of scan planes have become important in the routine practice of abdominal ultrasound. Different authors have defined the number and nomenclature of these "standard views" and the corresponding transducer placements differently. The most frequently described abdominal scans are shown in Figure 1.**7.**

Transducer movements

Once you have grasped the basics of transducer placement, you should become familiar with the basic patterns of transducer movement. Position the transducer for an upper abdominal transverse scan. The transducer can now be moved according to the patterns shown in Figure 1.**8**.

Perform each of these movements with the transducer, sticking closely to the patterns indicated for the time being. In an actual examination, of course, you would generally use various combinations of these patterns, but the beginner often encounters problems by using unintended or unwanted combinations of transducer movements. You should always be aware of the movements that you are making with the transducer.

There are five basic ways to move the transducer on the skin surface: sliding it on the flat, sliding it on edge, angling, rocking, and rotation.

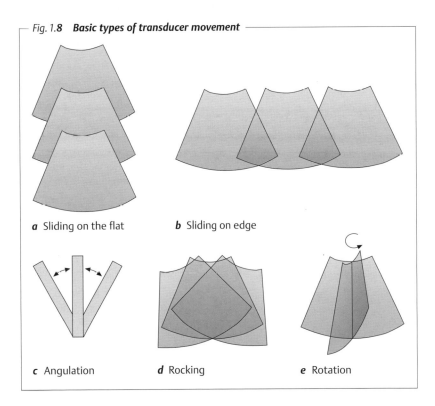

Fig. 1.8 **Basic types of transducer movement**

a Sliding on the flat   *b* Sliding on edge

c Angulation   *d* Rocking   *e* Rotation

Sliding on the flat. When you move the transducer across the skin with the flat side leading, you obtain a series of parallel scans that you can easily relate to one another during the examination. This is the easiest way to create a three-dimensional spatial impression from a set of two-dimensional slices. The beginner should make a special effort to keep the scans parallel to one another. Frequently, the sliding movement is combined with unwanted angulation of the probe. We can illustrate this with an example. Position the transducer for an upper abdominal longitudinal scan. Move the transducer laterally, keeping it at a constant vertical angle, while watching the image on the screen. You will obtain parallel sagittal sections (Fig. 1.**9a**). Now repeat this movement but keep the transducer perpendicular to the body surface. Notice that the transducer starts in a sagittal plane but ends up in a coronal plane because you have added angulation to the lateral movement (Fig. 1.**9b**).

Fig. 1.9 **Sliding the transducer on the flat, with and without angulation**

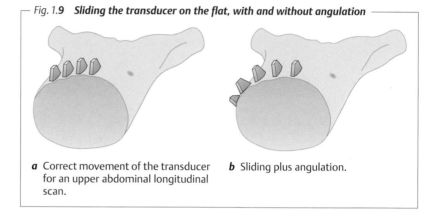

a Correct movement of the transducer for an upper abdominal longitudinal scan.

b Sliding plus angulation.

Sliding on edge. When you move the transducer across the skin with the narrow edge leading, you extend the field of view without leaving the initial scan plane. As a result, this maneuver does not provide a three-dimensional impression but an extended two-dimensional view (Fig. 1.**10a**). This movement is often combined with unintended rocking of the probe (Fig. 1.**10b**).

Fig. 1.10 **Sliding the transducer on the flat, with and without a rocking motion**

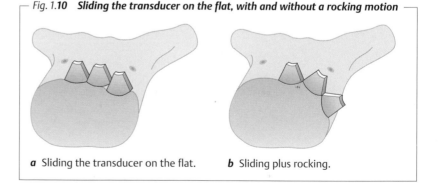

a Sliding the transducer on the flat.

b Sliding plus rocking.

Angling. Angling (tilting) the transducer produces a series of fan-shaped scans. This movement can give a good three-dimensional impression of the scanned anatomy, but extreme tilting of the probe can make spatial visualization difficult, as illustrated in Fig. 1.**11**. This type of section can be extremely difficult for a beginner to interpret during the examination.

Fig. 1.11
Angling the transducer.
Section 1 is a standard transverse scan, with the examiner looking up into the body from below. Section 2 is an oblique scan, which the examiner is viewing at a more posterior angle. Section 3 is almost in a coronal plane. The examiner is viewing this section from behind, so that the body is projected "upside down."

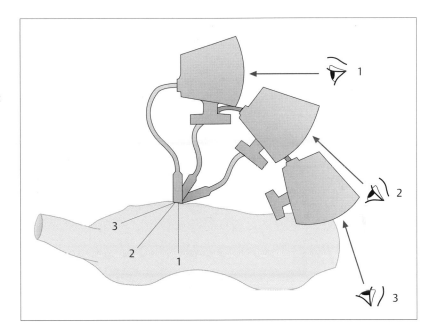

Angling the transducer is a useful technique for making narrow sweeps and for scanning through acoustic windows to avoid barriers located near the transducer.

Rocking. This movement, like sliding the transducer on edge, keeps to the initial scan plane and does not convey a three-dimensional impression. However, it can extend the field of view when scanning through a narrow acoustic window.

Rotation. Rotation is usually combined with a sliding movement of the transducer. It is useful for obtaining a continuous view of curved anatomic structures.

Isolated transducer rotation, in which the probe is turned about its central axis, can be used to demonstrate a structure in a second plane. For example, a vascular segment will appear circular in transverse section but elongated in the second plane, whereas a cyst will appear circular in both planes.

2 Basic Physical and Technical Principles

You now know how to adjust the ultrasound machine, how to optimize the image quality, and how to use the transducer. You are ready to begin scanning.

If you like, you may skip the following section and return to it later if you need to. It provides a brief review of the basic physical and technical principles of diagnostic ultrasound.

LEARNING GOALS

➤ Understand the production, propagation, and detection of ultrasound.
➤ Learn the differences between A-mode, B-mode, and M-mode scanning.
➤ Be able to recognize and distinguish artifacts.

Ultrasound

Definitions

Sound is a mechanical wave that travels longitudinally through an elastic medium.

Ultrasound is sound at a frequency beyond the range of human hearing. The frequency range of diagnostic ultrasound is between 1 and 20 MHz.

Propagation of sound

Reflection and refraction

When sound encounters a boundary between two media of different densities, some of the sound "bounces" back toward the source as an echo. The angle of incidence of the sound is equal to the angle at which the echo is returned. This phenomenon is called reflection. The rest of the sound continues to travel through the second medium but is deflected from its original path. This phenomenon is called refraction.

Impedance

Acoustic impedance is the measure of resistance to the propagation of sound waves. It is the product of the density of a medium and the velocity of sound in the medium. When there is a large difference in acoustic impedance between two adjacent media, a large portion of the sound will be reflected at the interface between the media.

Absorption

As a sound wave propagates through matter, some of its energy is converted by friction into heat. This loss of sound energy is called absorption.

Scatter

Besides reflection and refraction, scatter is another phenomenon that is important in the propagation of ultrasound. When ultrasound waves encounter a nonhomogeneous medium or a "rough" surface, a small part of their energy is scattered away from the object, in random directions, while most of the sound continues to propagate. In diagnostic ultrasound, some of this scattered sound is radiated back toward the transducer and contributes to image formation.

Production and detection of ultrasound waves: the pulse-echo principle

KEY POINT

The piezoelectric crystals in a transducer emit sound pulses and also receive the echoes.

Diagnostic ultrasound is based on the pulse-echo principle. The smallest functional unit of the ultrasound transducer is the piezoelectric crystal. This crystal has the property of converting electrical oscillations into mechanical vibrations, and vice versa. Thus, when the crystal is exposed to an alternating electric current, it will undergo mechanical deformation and generate sound waves. Conversely, when sound waves strike the crystal, they deform it and cause it to generate electrical impulses. One crystal can perform both functions in an alternating fashion.

First the piezoelectric crystal is exposed to an alternating electrical field, causing it to vibrate. The transducer emits a short, intense burst (pulse) of sound. Immediately thereafter, the transducer switches to the "listening" mode. The echoes reflected from different interfaces successively return to the crystal and cause it to vibrate. These vibrations are converted to electrical impulses, which are used to reconstruct an image.

Diagnostic ultrasound: propagation of ultrasound in biological tissue

From an ultrasound standpoint, the human body is composed of three basic materials: gas, soft tissues, and bone (Table 2.**1**).

Table 2.**1** Sound velocity (V), density (ρ) and impedance (Z = ρ × V) in various materials

Material	V (m/s)	ρ (g/cm³)	Z = ρ × V
Air	331	0.0012	41.3×10^{-5}
Tissue – Fat – Muscle – Liver – Water	1476 – 1570	0.928 – 1055	1.37 – 1.66
Bone	3 360	1.85	6.2

(after Dobrinski and Kremer)

The very large difference in acoustic impedance that exists between air and tissue ("impedance mismatch") causes 100% of the sound to be reflected at air/tissue interfaces. The impedance mismatch between bone and tissue is large enough to cause almost all of the sound to be reflected. The portion that continues to travel across the bone/tissue interface is too small to be utilized diagnostically. The small impedance mismatch that exists between different soft tissues is the basis for diagnostic ultrasound. Most of the sound waves are not reflected from the initial tissues layers and are available for scanning the deeper layers.

Producing an Image

KEY POINT

Two types of data — time and echo intensity — are used to make the acoustic signals visible in the A-mode, B-mode, and M-mode displays.

The detection of the returning sound pulses supplies two critical types of information:
➤ The time that it takes for the echo to reach the receiver. This determines the location of the reflecting interface in the monitor image.
➤ The intensity of the echo. This depends on the difference in hardness at the interface between the adjacent sound-conducting media.

A-Mode

A stands for "amplitude." The A-mode principle is as follows: A short ultrasound pulse is emitted and propagates through the tissue. The reflected echoes are displayed on a graph as vertical deflections along a time axis. The location of the deflections depends on the echo transit time, and their amplitude (height) depends on the intensity of the echoes.

B-Mode

B stands for "brightness." In the B-mode, the returning echoes are displayed as shades of gray rather than deflections along a baseline. The echo amplitude is represented by a gray level ranging from black to white. Each signal that is received along an image line is displayed as a one-dimensional gray-scale spot, and the individual image lines are briefly stored. The acoustic axis of the transducer is swept through the tissues to acquire the total number of lines needed to make a sectional image. All of the image lines are then accessed and assembled on the monitor to create a two-dimensional B-mode image.

M-Mode

M stands for "motion." The M-mode is used to display moving structures. As in B-mode, a gray-scale-modulated image line is produced. However, whereas the acoustic axis is moved in the two-dimensional B-mode display to acquire a large number of image lines, the acoustic axis in the M-mode display does not move. Instead, the same B-mode image line is displayed along a moving time base to graph the changing location of the mobile anatomic structures.

Fig. 2.1
A-mode, B-mode, and M-mode.
Shown for an acoustic axis through the heart.

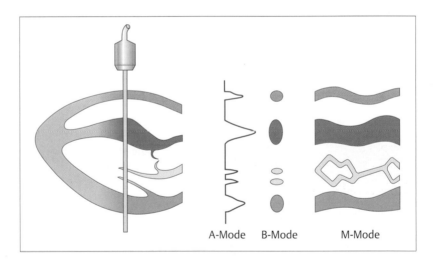

Figure 2.1 shows an ultrasound beam crossing multiple interfaces and undergoing partial reflection at each interface. In A-mode, the location of an amplitude spike corresponds to the location of the interface, and the height of the spike is proportional to the echo intensity. In B-mode, the amplitude of the echo is represented by the gray level of the spot. The image line is still one-dimensional, and a number of adjacent lines must be assembled to create the familiar two-dimensional B-mode image. M-mode also utilizes the gray-scale B-mode image line, but the acoustic axis remains stationary. The motion of reflective interfaces along the acoustic axis, as in the heart, alters the location of the signals displayed along the image line. Moving the recording paper creates a two-dimensional graphic record that documents the motion of the interfaces over time.

Artifacts

Artifacts in the ultrasound image are echoes that do not correspond to an anatomic structure. They result from the physical properties of ultrasound propagation in tissues.

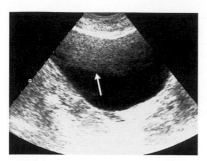

Fig. 2.2
Noise. Scan through the urinary bladder. Myriad fine internal echoes (↑) are seen within the part of the bladder that is closest to the transducer.

Noise

Noise refers to the appearance of grainy echoes, especially in the proximal portion of cystic areas (Fig. 2.2). It is caused mainly by excessive gain in the near field. Noise can be reduced by lowering the gain setting.

Acoustic shadowing

An acoustic shadow is an echo-free area located behind an insonated structure (Fig. 2.3). It is caused by total reflection (e.g., by air) or absorption (bone, gallstones) of the sound energy.

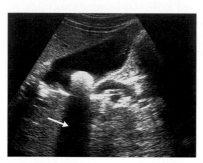

Fig. 2.3
Acoustic shadow. This artifact appears as an echo-free streak behind a gallstone (→).

Posterior acoustic enhancement

In posterior acoustic enhancement, the area behind an echo-free structure appears more echogenic than its surroundings (Fig. 2.4). When the sound passes through the echo-free structure, typically a cyst, it undergoes very little energy loss and attenuation. Because of this, the area behind the cyst appears brighter in relation to the surrounding tissues. The term "enhancement" is somewhat misleading, as this phenomenon is actually due to decreased attenuation.

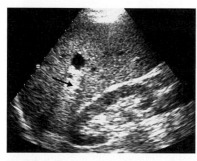

Fig. 2.4
Posterior acoustic enhancement. This artifact forms an echogenic streak in the liver tissue behind a cyst (→).

Reverberations

Reverberations occur in two typical forms: parallel bands of echoes spaced at equal intervals (Fig. 2.5a) and a line of echoes resembling a comet tail (Fig. 2.5b). Reverberations occur at the interfaces of adjacent media that differ greatly in their acoustic impedance. The ultrasound waves are partially reflected from the second interface, and some of these echoes are reflected again from the back of the first interface. This sets up repetitive back-and-forth reflections that either appear as distinct parallel bands (first form) or, at very strong reflectors, blend into a narrow streak resembling a comet tail (second form, also called a comet-tail artifact).

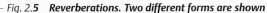

Fig. 2.5 Reverberations. Two different forms are shown

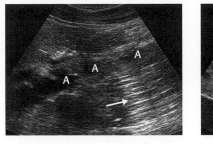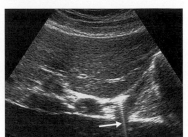

a Parallel artifacts (→). These are produced by the highly reflective vessel walls in a tangential longitudinal scan through the aortic wall (A).

b Comet-tail artifact. Very fine, parallel reverberations behind the gas-containing duodenum blend into a streak resembling a comet tail (→).

Beam-width artifact

The beam-width artifact (section-thickness artifact) appears as a collection of fine, grainy echoes distributed along the inside of cystic structures whose wall is struck obliquely by the ultrasound beam (Fig. 2.**6**). The main beam emitted by the transducer has a definite width. When the beam encounters an oblique interface, the beam width overlaps both the echo-free interior of the cyst and its highly reflective wall. Because the echogenicities of these different structures are averaged together electronically to form an image, smudgy echoes appear to line the cyst wall (pseudosludge).

Fig. 2.6 Beam-width artifact

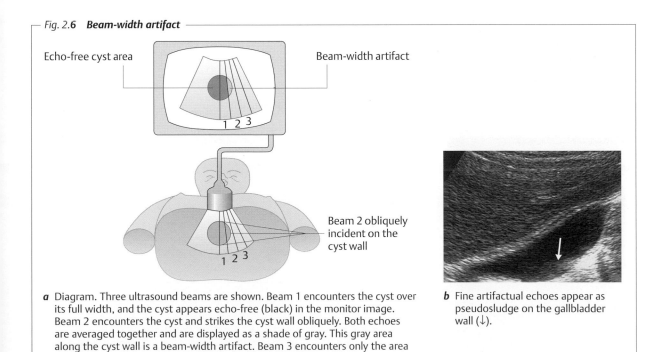

a Diagram. Three ultrasound beams are shown. Beam 1 encounters the cyst over its full width, and the cyst appears echo-free (black) in the monitor image. Beam 2 encounters the cyst and strikes the cyst wall obliquely. Both echoes are averaged together and are displayed as a shade of gray. This gray area along the cyst wall is a beam-width artifact. Beam 3 encounters only the area outside the cyst, which appears dense and bright on the monitor.

b Fine artifactual echoes appear as pseudosludge on the gallbladder wall (↓).

Echo-free cyst area

Beam-width artifact

Beam 2 obliquely incident on the cyst wall

Side-lobe artifact

Side-lobe artifacts are bright, curved lines that are usually seen in hypoechoic or echo-free structures (Fig. 2.**7**). They are caused by side lobes, which are secondary oblique concentrations of energy located off the main beam axis. When the echo from a side lobe reaches the receiver with sufficient energy, it is assigned to the main beam and is therefore displayed at a false location. Due to the low energy of the side lobe, a strong reflector (e.g., air) and hypoechoic or echo-free surroundings (gallbladder, large vessels) must be present in order for the artifact to be seen.

*Fig. 2.***7**   *Side-lobe artifact*

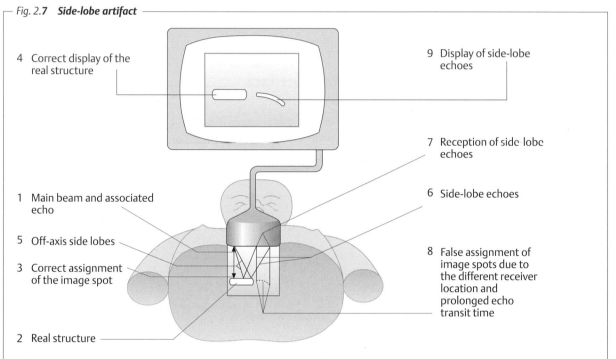

4 Correct display of the real structure

9 Display of side-lobe echoes

7 Reception of side-lobe echoes

1 Main beam and associated echo

6 Side-lobe echoes

5 Off-axis side lobes

3 Correct assignment of the image spot

8 False assignment of image spots due to the different receiver location and prolonged echo transit time

2 Real structure

a Diagram. Side-lobe echoes cause the image spots to be displayed at a false location.

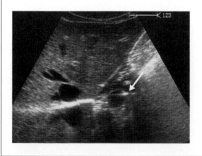

b Side-lobe echoes from the spinal column produce a curved streak (↓) in the vena cava.

Mirror-image artifact

A mirror-image artifact is the virtual image of a real object that forms behind a highly reflective interface (Fig. 2.**8**). It is caused by deflection of the beam at the "specular" reflector. The virtual image appears behind the interface in the path of the main beam.

Fig. 2.**8** *Mirror-image artifact*

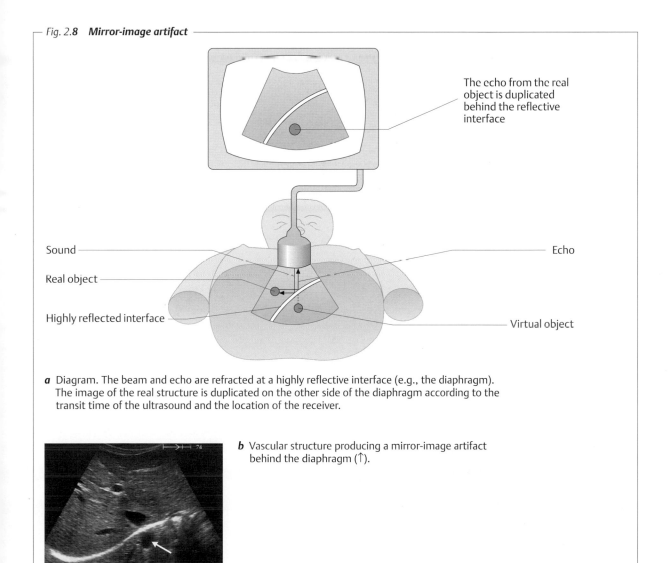

The echo from the real object is duplicated behind the reflective interface

Sound

Echo

Real object

Highly reflected interface

Virtual object

a Diagram. The beam and echo are refracted at a highly reflective interface (e.g., the diaphragm). The image of the real structure is duplicated on the other side of the diaphragm according to the transit time of the ultrasound and the location of the receiver.

b Vascular structure producing a mirror-image artifact behind the diaphragm (↑).

Lateral edge shadow

A lateral edge shadow is a thin acoustic shadow that appears distal to the lateral edges of a cystic structure (Fig. 2.**9**). It is caused by the refraction and scattering of sound striking the cyst wall at a tangential angle. Due to the energy loss that occurs, the sound does not propagate to deeper levels, and an acoustic shadow is formed.

*Fig. 2.**9** Lateral edge shadows*

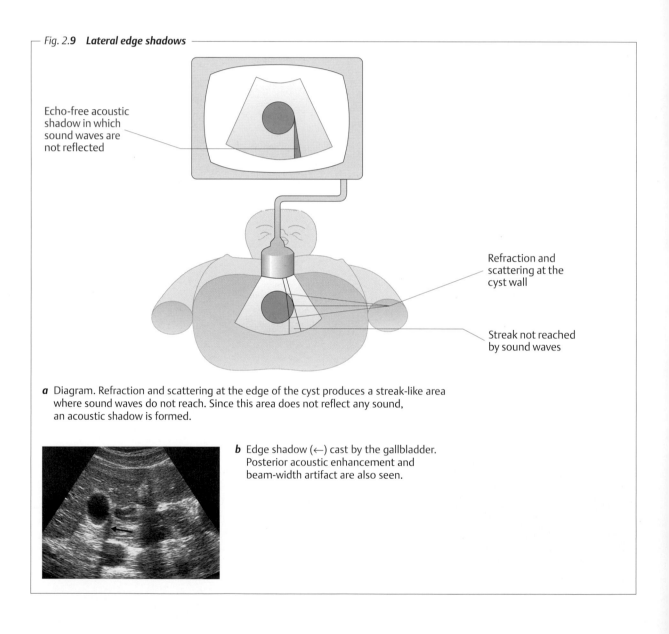

Echo-free acoustic shadow in which sound waves are not reflected

Refraction and scattering at the cyst wall

Streak not reached by sound waves

a Diagram. Refraction and scattering at the edge of the cyst produces a streak-like area where sound waves do not reach. Since this area does not reflect any sound, an acoustic shadow is formed.

b Edge shadow (←) cast by the gallbladder. Posterior acoustic enhancement and beam-width artifact are also seen.

Blood Vessels: The Aorta and its Branches, the Vena cava and its Tributaries

Organ Boundaries

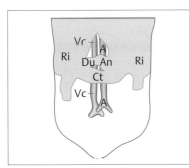

Fig. 3.1
Barriers to scanning the aorta (A) and vena cava (Vc).
The transverse colon (Ct) is a barrier to scanning, along with the antrum (An) and duodenum (Du). Ri = costal arch.

LEARNING GOALS

➤ Locate and identify the aorta and vena cava.
➤ Demonstrate the aorta and vena cava in their entirety.

The aorta and vena cava run parallel, anterior, and slightly lateral to the spinal column in the retroperitoneum. Just below the diaphragm, the vena cava initially is slightly more anterior than the aorta and is surrounded predominantly by the liver. The aorta is covered by the esophagogastric junction as it pierces the diaphragm and is more difficult to image than the vena cava (Fig. 3.1).

Locating the aorta and vena cava

Barriers to scanning

The two main barriers to scanning the aorta and vena cava are the stomach and transverse colon.

Optimizing the scanning conditions

Usually the two vessels can be quickly located by sliding the transducer across the upper abdomen.

Organ identification

Start with the transducer placed transversely in the midline of the upper abdomen below the xiphoid. From there you can almost always image the aorta and vena cava in transverse section by angling the transducer slightly up (cephalad) and down (caudad), as shown in Fig. 3.2.

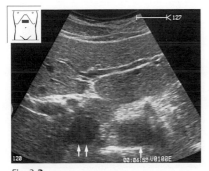

Fig. 3.2
Upper abdominal transverse scan of the aorta and vena cava.
Aorta (↑), vena cava (↑↑).

Demonstrating the aorta and vena cava in their entirety

Demonstrating the aorta and vena cava in transverse section

Define both vessels in an upper abdominal transverse section and scan slowly down the length of the vessels to the level of the bifurcation (Fig. 3.**3**). It is normal for your view to be obscured intermittently by bowel gas, mainly in the transverse colon.

Fig. 3.3   *Transverse scans of the aorta and vena cava*

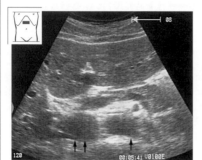 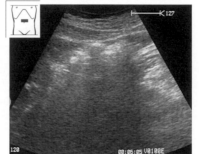 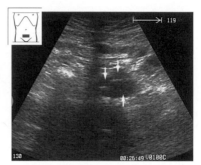

a Transverse scan between the umbilicus and xiphoid. Aorta (↑), vena cava (↑↑).

b Transverse scan just above the umbilicus. Details are obscured by gas in the transverse colon.

c Transverse scan at the level of the bifurcation. Aortic bifurcation (↓↓), vena cava (↑).

Demonstrating the aorta and vena cava in longitudinal section

While watching the screen, rotate the transducer over the aorta in the upper abdomen from a transverse to a longitudinal plane of section. As you move the transducer slowly toward the right side, the aorta will disappear and the vena cava will come into view (Fig. 3.**4**). Scan across the entire aorta and vena cava. Repeat this pass several times.

Fig. 3.4   *Upper abdominal longitudinal scans of the aorta and vena cava*

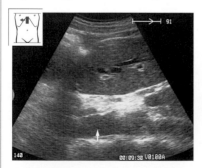 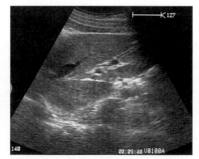 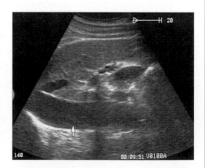

a Longitudinal scan of the aorta (↑) demonstrating the entry of the aorta into the thoracic cavity.

b The transducer was moved to the right. This scan cuts the space between the aorta and vena cava.

c The transducer was moved farther to the right, defining the vena cava in longitudinal section (↑).

Now move the transducer down to the midabdomen. You will notice that the vessels are obscured by gas — usually in the transverse colon, which is cut transversely by the scan plane. As before, scan slowly across the entire aorta and vena cava several times (Fig. 3.**5**).

Fig. 3.**5** *Midabdominal longitudinal scans of the aorta and vena cava*

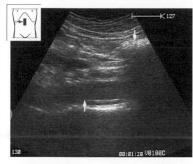
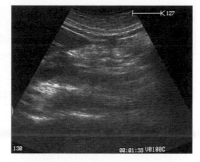
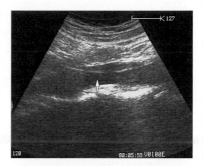

a Longitudinal scan of the aorta (↑). Gas is visible in the transverse colon (↓).

b The transducer was moved to the right. This scan cuts the space between the aorta and vena cava.

c The transducer was moved farther to the right, showing a longitudinal section of the vena cava (↑).

Abnormalities in the course of the aorta

Elongation and kinking of the aorta may occur with ageing (Fig. 3.**6**). In these cases only small segments of the kinked aorta can be seen in longitudinal sections. In transverse sections, you will see the lumen deviate toward the right or left side as you scan down the vessel.

Fig. 3.**6** *Kinking of the aorta toward the left side*

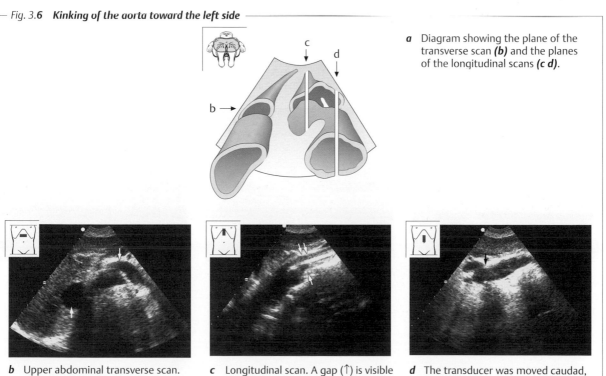

a Diagram showing the plane of the transverse scan (**b**) and the planes of the longitudinal scans (**c d**).

b Upper abdominal transverse scan. A = aorta kinked to the left (↓), vena cava (↑).

c Longitudinal scan. A gap (↑) is visible below the superior mesenteric artery (↓↓).

d The transducer was moved caudad, demonstrating the continuation of the aorta and a posterior kink in the vessel (↓).

Organ Details

KEY POINTS

The aorta cannot be compressed with the transducer.

The diameter of the aorta gently tapers from 2.5 cm superiorly to 2.0 cm inferiorly.

The lumen of the vena cava becomes smaller during inspiration.

Demonstrating arterial and venous pulsations

Demonstrate the aorta in an upper abdominal longitudinal scan. Notice the firm beat of its pulsations. Now image the vena cava in longitudinal section and observe the soft, double-beat pattern of its pulsations.

Evaluating the vessel walls and lumina

Image the aorta in longitudinal section. Look at its thick, echogenic wall. Occasionally a typical three-layered wall structure can be seen (Fig. 3.**7**). Note how the size of its lumen does not change during pulsations or during inspiration/expiration. Apply pressure over the aorta with the transducer and notice that it is not compressible. The normal aorta tapers from above downward, its diameter decreasing from approximately 2.5 cm to 2.0 cm.

Define the vena cava in longitudinal section. Notice its thin wall and the changes in its caliber during the pulse phases. Have the subject breathe in and out (Figs. 3.**8**, 3.**9**) and observe how the lumen narrows during inspiration.

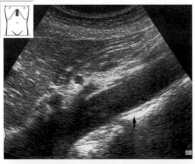

Fig. 3.7 Longitudinal scan of the aorta. The three-layered wall structure is faintly visible (↑). Notice the smooth outline of the vessel wall.

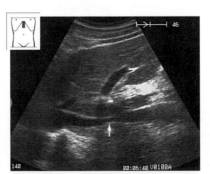

Fig. 3.8 Longitudinal scan of the vena cava during inspiration (↑).

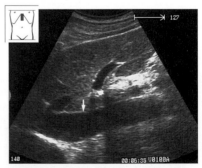

Fig. 3.9 Vena cava during expiration (↓).

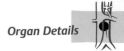

Abnormalities of the aortic wall and lumen

Atherosclerotic plaque. It is common to find atherosclerotic plaques on the inner wall of the aorta and its branches (Figs. 3.**10** – 3.**13**).

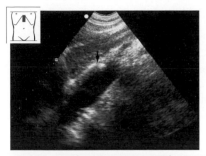

Fig. 3.10   Atherosclerotic plaque (↓) at the origin of the celiac trunk in longitudinal section.

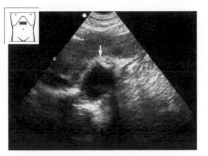

Fig. 3.11   Transverse scan at the level of the plaque (↓). Same patient as in Fig. 3.**10**.

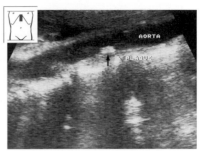

Fig. 3.12   Atherosclerotic plaque on the posterior wall of the aorta (↑).

Aortic aneurysm. Most aortic aneurysms occur at an infrarenal level, and generally they are easy to detect. A saccular aneurysm (Fig. 3.**14**) appears as a circumscribed, asymmetrical outpouching of the aorta, while a fusiform aneurysm (Fig. 3.**15**) uniformly affects the circumference of the vessel (Fig. 3.**16**). With a dissecting aneurysm, the intimal flap can be recognized as a bright echo (Fig. 3.**17**). Table 3.**1** reviews the sonographic features of aortic aneurysm.

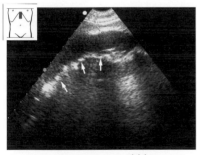

Fig. 3.13   Atherosclerosis (↑↑↑) involving a long segment of the aortic posterior wall.

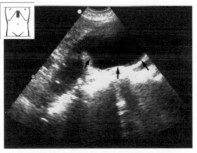

Fig. 3.14   Saccular aortic aneurysm (↑↑↑).

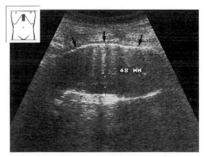

Fig. 3.15   Fusiform aortic aneurysm (↓↓↓).

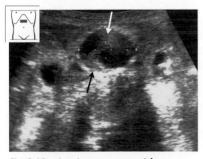

Fig. 3.16   Aortic aneurysm with a thrombus. Notice the mural thrombus (↑↓) and two lumina.

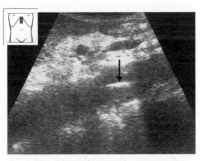

Fig. 3.17   Dissecting aortic aneurysm. The echogenic intima (↓) is clearly defined.

Table 3.**1**   Sonographic features of aortic aneurysm

Distension > 30 mm
Pulsations
Signs of aortic sclerosis
Possible partial thrombosis

Aortic aneurysms tend to enlarge over time. The larger the aneurysm, the more rapid its progression. Aneurysms less than 5 cm in diameter grow by 2 – 4 mm each year. Cases of this kind should be scanned every three months to evaluate size. Aneurysms with a diameter of 5 cm or more grow by up to 6 mm per year. These cases should be evaluated for surgical treatment. With aneurysms larger than 7 cm, the risk of rupture in one year is greater than 50%.

Luminal and wall abnormalities of the vena cava

Heart failure. Scanning in patients with overt right heart failure demonstrates an enlarged vena cava (> 2 cm) that is resistant to compression and does not change its caliber with respiration (Fig. 3.**18**).

Vena cava thrombosis. A thrombus appears as an intraluminal area of high echogenicity (Fig. 3.**19**). As in heart failure, the vessel does not show caliber changes with respiration. Table 3.**2** lists the sonographic features of vena cava thrombosis.

Table 3.**2** Sonographic features of vena cava thrombosis

Distension

Lack of compressibility

Intraluminal echogenicity

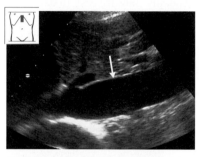

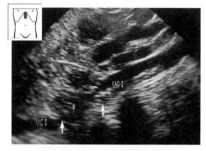

*Fig. 3.**18** Right-sided heart failure.* Ultrasound shows an enlarged, noncompressible vena cava (↓) 2.9 cm in diameter.

*Fig. 3.**19** Vena cava thrombosis (↑).* The lumen is occluded by echogenic thrombus.

Identifying and defining the branches of the aorta and vena cava

Aortic branches

You know the anatomy of the aortic branches that can be seen with ultrasound: the celiac trunk with the hepatic artery, splenic artery, and left gastric artery; the superior mesenteric artery; the right and left renal arteries; and finally the right and left iliac arteries (Table 3.**3**). These structures create patterns in longitudinal and transverse scans that, ideally, can be used as landmarks (Fig. 3.**20**).

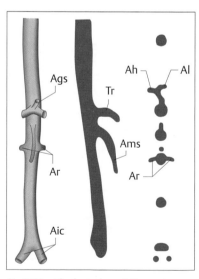

*Fig. 3.**20** The branches of the aorta viewed from the front, from the side, and in cross section.*
Tr = celiac trunk, Ah = hepatic artery, Al = splenic artery, Ags = left gastric artery, Ams = superior mesenteric artery, Aic = common iliac arteries, Ar = renal artery

Table 3.**3**   Branches of the abdominal aorta

Parietal	Visceral
Lumbar arteries	Celiac trunk
Common iliac arteries	– Left gastric artery
	– Hepatic artery
	– Splenic artery
	Superior mesenteric artery
	Renal arteries
	Inferior mesenteric artery

Demonstrating the aortic branches

Place the transducer longitudinally in the epigastrium. Identify the celiac trunk and the superior mesenteric artery (Fig. 3.**21 a**). Rotate the transducer under vision to a transverse plane and identify the celiac trunk in cross section (Fig. 3.**21 b**). Now scan transversely down the aorta, identifying the origin of the superior mesenteric artery and its course anterior to the aorta (Fig. 3.**21 c, d**).

Fig. 3.21   **Demonstrating the celiac trunk and superior mesenteric artery**

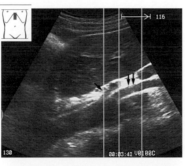

a   High longitudinal scan of the aorta, demonstrating the celiac trunk (→) and superior mesenteric artery (↓↓). Lines indicate the transverse scan planes in *b*, *c*, and *d*.

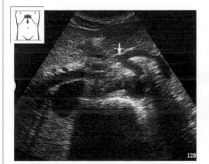

b   Transverse scan at the level of the celiac trunk (↓).

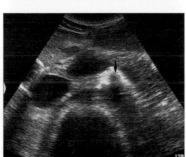

c   Transverse scan at the level of the origin of the superior mesenteric artery (↓).

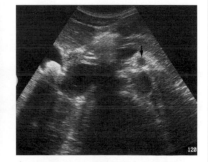

d   Transverse scan at the level of the aorta and superior mesenteric artery (↓).

Position the transducer for a slightly lower longitudinal scan (Fig. 3.**22a**), then rotate it to a transverse scan. Identify the origin of the renal arteries, scan down the aortic segment below that, and continue scanning to the level of the bifurcation (Fig. 3.**22b–d**).

Fig. 3.22   Demonstrating the renal arteries and aortic bifurcation

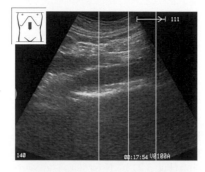

a   Low longitudinal scan of the aorta. Lines indicate the transverse scan planes in *b*, *c*, and *d*.

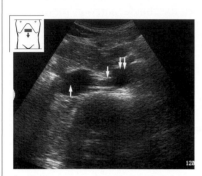

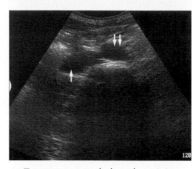

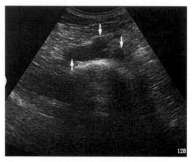

b   Transverse scan at the level of the renal arteries (↓). Aorta (↓↓), vena cava (↑).

c   Transverse scan below the origin of the renal arteries. Aorta (↓↓), vena cava (↑).

d   Transverse scan at the level of the bifurcation. The iliac vessels (↓) are seen. Vena cava (↑).

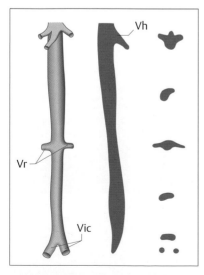

*Fig. 3.23   **Tributaries of the inferior vena cava** viewed from the front, from the side, and in cross section. Vh = hepatic vein, Vr = renal veins, Vic = common iliac veins.. Vh = hepatic vein, Vr = renal veins, Vic = common iliac veins.*

Vena cava tributaries

You know the tributaries of the inferior vena cava that are visible with ultrasound: the hepatic veins, renal veins, and iliac veins. These vessels also have typical ultrasound appearances (Fig. 3.**23**).

Demonstrating the vena cava tributaries

Place the transducer longitudinally over the upper part of the inferior vena cava. Angle the scan through the upper portion of the liver, and identify the vena cava at the site where it pierces the diaphragm (Fig. 3.**24a**). Now rotate the transducer to a transverse plane and locate the site where the hepatic veins enter the vena cava below the diaphragm (Fig. 3.**24b**). Move the scan down the vena cava and observe the course of the hepatic veins through the periphery of the liver, then the distal segment of the vena cava itself (Fig. 3.**24c, d**).

Fig. 3.**24** **Demonstrating the hepatic veins**

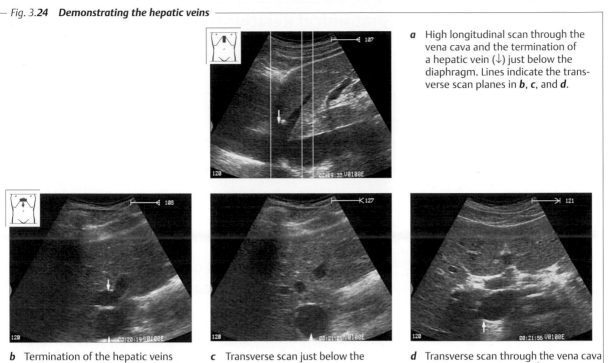

a High longitudinal scan through the vena cava and the termination of a hepatic vein (↓) just below the diaphragm. Lines indicate the transverse scan planes in *b*, *c*, and *d*.

b Termination of the hepatic veins in cross section (↓). Vena cava (↑).

c Transverse scan just below the termination of the hepatic veins. Vena cava (↑).

d Transverse scan through the vena cava in the upper abdomen (↑).

Next, position the transducer for a low longitudinal scan and again identify the vena cava (Fig. 3.**25 a**). Rotate the transducer to a transverse plane and locate the terminations of the renal veins (Fig. 3.**25 b**). Scan down to the level of the bifurcation (Fig. 3.**25 c, d**).

Fig. 3.**25** **Demonstrating the renal veins**

a Low longitudinal scan through the vena cava (Vc). Lines indicate the transverse scan planes in *b*, *c*, and *d*.

b Transverse scan at the level of the renal veins (↓). A = aorta, Vc = vena cava, Ams = superior mesenteric artery.

c Transverse scan above the bifurcation.

d Transverse scan at the level of the bifurcation (↓↓).

Anatomical Relationships

LEARNING GOALS

➤ Clearly demonstrate the relationships of the aorta and vena cava to the diaphragm, liver, and gastric cardia.
➤ Clearly define the aortic branches and vena cava tributaries and their course.

The vessels of the retroperitoneum are easily to identify with ultrasound, making them useful landmarks for scanning. You should make an effort to become familiar with them.

Relationship of the aorta and vena cava to the diaphragm, liver, and cardia

Position the transducer for an upper abdominal transverse scan and identify the liver, which at this level is interposed between the aorta and vena cava. The cardioesophageal junction lies anterior to the aorta. The hypoechoic musculature of the diaphragm is also seen (Fig. 3.**26a**). Rotate the transducer to a longitudinal plane and scan through the region. Identify the vena cava (Fig. 3.**26b**), the caudate lobe of the liver (Fig. 3.**26c**), the aorta, and the gastric cardia lying anterior to it (Fig. 3.**26d**). (The caudate lobe is described in detail on p. 67 ff. and the gastroesophageal junction on p. 166 ff.)

─ *Fig. 3.26   The relationship of the aorta and vena cava to the diaphragm, liver, and cardia* ─

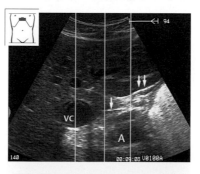

a Transverse scan of the aorta (A) and vena cava (Vc) just below the diaphragm. Crus of diaphragm (↓), gastroesophageal junction (↓↓). Lines indicate the longitudinal scan planes in *b*, *c*, and *d*.

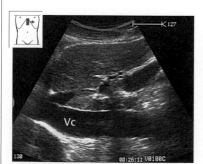

b Longitudinal scan through the vena cava (Vc).

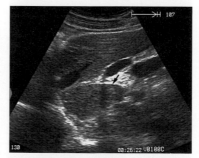

c Longitudinal scan through the caudate lobe (↓).

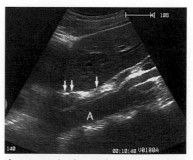

d Longitudinal scan through the aorta (A). Note also the diaphragm crus (↓) and the gastroesophageal junction (↓↓).

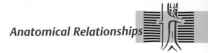

Area surrounding the celiac trunk and the course of the hepatic artery, splenic artery, and left gastric artery

The common hepatic artery curves upward and to the right from the celiac trunk to the porta hepatis, where it is accompanied by the portal vein and bile duct. The splenic artery turns to the left and runs with the splenic vein to the hilum of the spleen. This artery takes a very tortuous course. The left gastric artery passes upward from the celiac trunk and usually can be traced only a short distance (Figs. 3.**27**, 3.**28**).

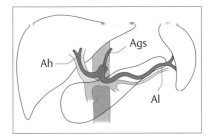

Fig. 3.27 The celiac trunk and its branches, viewed from the front.
Notice that the hepatic artery (Ah) and splenic artery (Al) initially curve downward from their origin at the celiac trunk before passing toward the liver and spleen. Aqs = left gastric artery.

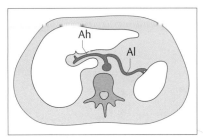

Fig. 3.28 Celiac trunk, hepatic artery, and splenic artery in cross section.
Notice that the celiac trunk is directed to the right and is continuous with the hepatic artery. The splenic artery first runs horizontally and then turns posteriorly and to the left.

Demonstrating the splenic artery, hepatic artery, and left gastric artery in longitudinal section

Sometimes you will see a phenomenon in longitudinal scans that may be somewhat confusing at first. It occurs when the scan simultaneously cuts the origin of the celiac trunk and the splenic artery anterior to it (Fig. 3.**29 a**). Figure 3.**29 b** explains this phenomenon.

Fig. 3.29 *Demonstrating the celiac trunk and splenic artery in longitudinal section*

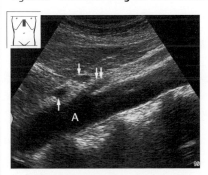

a Longitudinal scan through the aorta (A), celiac trunk (↑), splenic artery (↓), and superior mesenteric artery (↓↓).

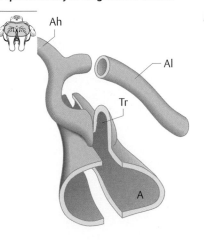

b Explanation of the phenomenon in *a*. The celiac trunk initially runs to the right and gives rise to the splenic artery, which courses to the left. This explains how a longitudinal scan can cut both vessels simultaneously.

Tr = celiac trunk
Ah = hepatic artery
Al = splenic artery
A   = aorta

Place the transducer longitudinally over the aorta, obtaining a sectional view of the celiac trunk (Fig. 3.**30a, b**). Mentally picture the splenic artery coursing behind the image plane. Now slide the transducer slowly to the left and follow the section of the splenic artery as it moves across the field of view (Fig. 3.**30c–e**).

Fig. 3.30 **Demonstrating the splenic artery in longitudinal section**

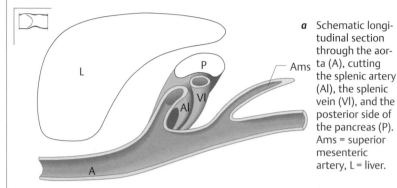

a Schematic longitudinal section through the aorta (A), cutting the splenic artery (Al), the splenic vein (Vl), and the posterior side of the pancreas (P). Ams = superior mesenteric artery, L = liver.

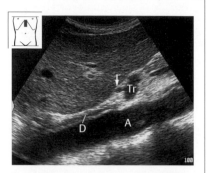

b Ultrasound image corresponding to **a**. You see the aorta (A), the anteriorly adjacent diaphragm crus (D), and the celiac trunk (Tr), from which the left gastric artery (↓) arises.

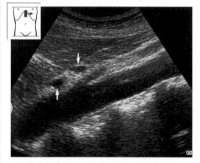

c The transducer was moved slightly to the left. This plane simultaneously cuts the celiac trunk (↑) and splenic artery (↓) (see also Fig. 3.**29**).

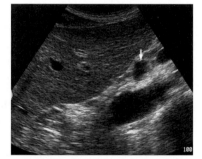

d The transducer was moved farther to the left. The aortic section gradually disappears, and the splenic artery (↓) is still seen.

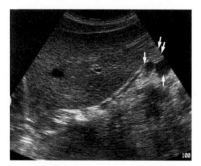

e Scanning farther to the left, the splenic artery (↓), splenic vein (↑), and pancreas (↓↓) can be identified on the right side of the image.

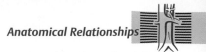
Bring the transducer back to its original position (Fig. 3.**31 a**) and then move it slowly to the right (Fig. 3.**31 b–d**). Observe the section of the hepatic artery, which is shown schematically in Fig. 3.**31 e**.

Fig. 3.31 **Demonstrating the hepatic artery in longitudinal section**

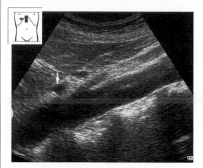

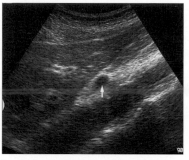

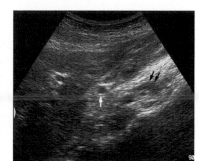

a Longitudinal scan through the aorta and celiac trunk (↓).

b The transducer was moved a short distance to the right. The aortic section narrows. The hepatic artery (↑) is seen.

c The transducer was moved farther to the right. The hepatic artery (↑) is still visible, and part of the confluence (↓↓) comes into view.

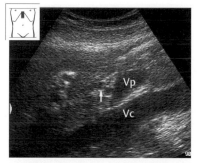

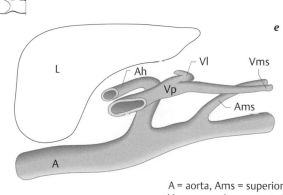

e Diagram corresponding to image *d*. Longitudinal section cuts across the hepatic artery (Ah) and portal vein (Vp). The further course of the vessels is located behind the plane of section.

d The transducer was moved still farther to the right. You see the hepatic artery (↑), portal vein (Vp), and also the vena cava (Vc).

A = aorta, Ams = superior mesenteric artery, Vms = superior mesenteric vein, Vl = splenic vein, L = liver

Demonstrating the hepatic artery and splenic artery in transverse section

The down-curved portions of the hepatic artery and splenic artery may occasionally cause peculiar imaging phenomena that are confusing initially. Refer back to Fig. 3.**27**. Both vessels show a marked downward curve as they leave the celiac trunk. Because of this, each artery may be cut twice in the same transverse plane — once at the origin and once in the periphery (Fig. 3.**32**). Figure 3.**33** shows the appearance of this phenomenon in actual images.

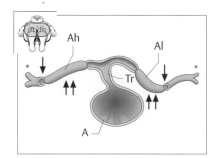

*Fig. 3.**32** **Cross section of the aorta and celiac trunk at the origins of the hepatic and splenic arteries.***
As you see, this plane of section cuts the arteries at their origins and also more peripherally (↓). The down-curved segments of both arteries (↑↑) lie in front of the image plane, and the peripheral segments passing to the porta hepatis and splenic hilum (*) are behind it.

A = aorta, Tr = celiac trunk,
Ah = hepatic artery,
Al = splenic artery

*Fig. 3.**33*** **Demonstrating the hepatic artery and splenic artery in transverse sections**

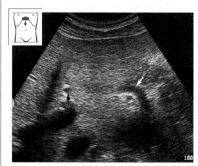

a High transverse scan cuts the peripheral portion of the hepatic artery (↑) and splenic artery (↓).

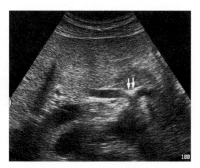

b Midlevel scan on the plane shown in Fig. 3.**32**. The bifurcation of the celiac trunk (↓↓) is seen.

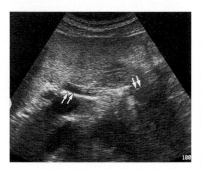

c Low transverse scan demonstrates portions of the hepatic artery (↑↑) and splenic artery (↓↓) that are outside the image plane in Fig. 3.**32**.

Superior mesenteric artery, splenic vein, and renal vessels

You are probably familiar with the frontal anatomy of these vessels. The splenic vein passes over the superior mesenteric artery. The renal vessels lie directly below the origin of the superior mesenteric artery. Their distance from the artery is variable, as is the course of the splenic vein (Fig. 3.**34a**). You may be less familiar with the cross-sectional anatomy of this region. Please note: the renal arteries are posterior and the renal veins are anterior. The left renal vein is physiologically compressed between the aorta and superior mesenteric artery and shows mild congestion on the left side, proximal to the compression site. The right renal artery compresses the vena cava from the posterior side (Fig. 3.**34b**). The diagram in Fig. 3.**34c** illustrates these relationships in a lateral oblique view.

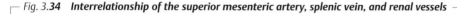
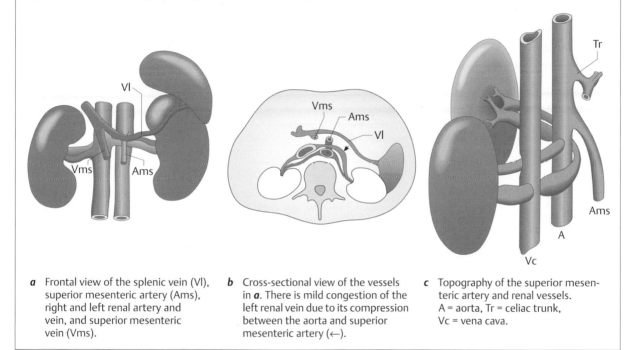

Fig. 3.**34** *Interrelationship of the superior mesenteric artery, splenic vein, and renal vessels*

a Frontal view of the splenic vein (Vl), superior mesenteric artery (Ams), right and left renal artery and vein, and superior mesenteric vein (Vms).

b Cross-sectional view of the vessels in *a*. There is mild congestion of the left renal vein due to its compression between the aorta and superior mesenteric artery (←).

c Topography of the superior mesenteric artery and renal vessels. A = aorta, Tr = celiac trunk, Vc = vena cava.

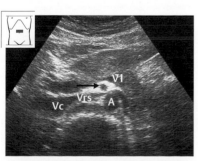

Fig. 3.**35** *The left right ventricle (Vrs) in transverse section.*
A = aorta, Vc = vena cava, Vl = splenic vein, superior mesenteric artery (→).

Demonstrating the superior mesenteric artery, splenic vein, and renal vessels in transverse section

Position the transducer for an upper abdominal transverse scan and locate the superior mesenteric artery and the splenic vein, which overlies the artery anteriorly. Now scan caudad in parallel sections. With some luck (which you will need), you can identify the left renal vein (Fig. 3.**35**); it runs to the left between the aorta and the superior mesenteric artery. Typically this vein is narrowed beneath the superior mesenteric artery and then expands on the left side of the aorta. Scan down through this region, spacing the scans at small intervals. When you know what to look for, you can frequently identify the renal arteries.

In many cases you can trace the right renal vessels back to the kidney. Place the probe transversely to the right of the midline and image the vena

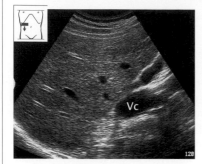

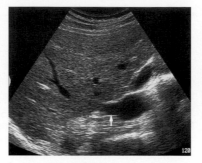

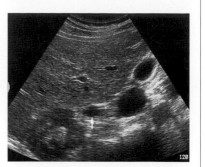

a Transverse scan above the kidney through the vena cava (Vc).

b Scan at a slightly lower level demonstrates the termination of the renal vein (↑).

c Scanning lower, the section of the renal vein approaches the renal hilum (↑).

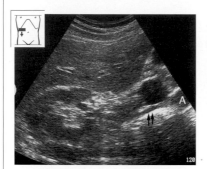

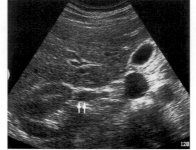

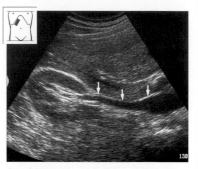

d Now the renal artery, which arises from the aorta (A), comes into view (↑↑).

e The sectioned artery moves closer to the kidney (↑↑).

f Oblique scan parallel to the costal arch defines the full length of the renal vein (↓↓↓).

cava (Fig. 3.**36a**). Starting from a plane above the level of the kidneys, slowly move the transducer caudad. If it is not hidden by bowel gas, you can recognize the termination of the large right renal vein (Fig. 3.**36b**). As you slide the transducer lower, the renal vein will appear to "detach" from the vena cava and move laterally toward the kidney. This occurs because the renal vein runs laterally downward at a slightly oblique angle. As the scan moves lower, the vein approaches the renal hilum (Fig. 3.**36c**). Usually the renal artery, which parallels the vein, will also come into view (Fig. 3.**36d, e**). An oblique scan parallel to the costal arch can define the full length of the renal vein (Fig. 3.**36f**). An analogous scanning technique on the left side is very rarely successful in defining the left renal vessels.

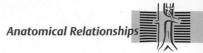

Demonstrating the renal vessels in longitudinal section

When you view the renal vessels in transverse section, you will see that there are five standard planes for imaging these vessels in longitudinal section (Fig. 3.**37**).

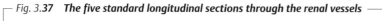

Fig. 3.37   *The five standard longitudinal sections through the renal vessels*

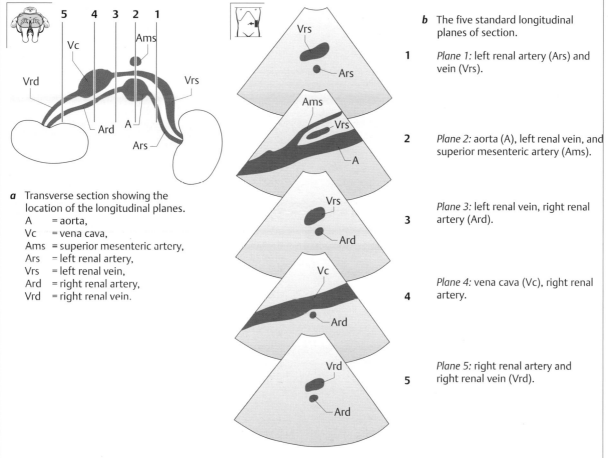

a Transverse section showing the location of the longitudinal planes.
A   = aorta,
Vc   = vena cava,
Ams   = superior mesenteric artery,
Ars   = left renal artery,
Vrs   = left renal vein,
Ard   = right renal artery,
Vrd   = right renal vein.

b The five standard longitudinal planes of section.

1 *Plane 1:* left renal artery (Ars) and vein (Vrs).

2 *Plane 2:* aorta (A), left renal vein, and superior mesenteric artery (Ams).

3 *Plane 3:* left renal vein, right renal artery (Ard).

4 *Plane 4:* vena cava (Vc), right renal artery.

5 *Plane 5:* right renal artery and right renal vein (Vrd).

Place the transducer longitudinally over the aorta and identify the aorta, the superior mesenteric artery, and the compressed left renal vein (Fig. 3.**38a, b**). Move the transducer to the left in small increments. Observe that the aorta disappears. Now locate the large anterior vein and small artery. You will not be able to track both vessels to the renal hilum (Fig. 3.**38c–e**).

Fig. 3.38 *Demonstrating the left renal vessels in longitudinal sections*

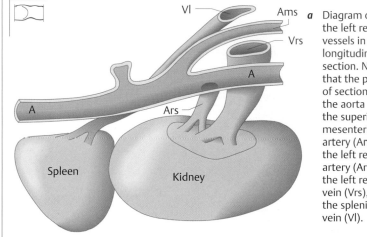

a Diagram of the left renal vessels in longitudinal section. Note that the plane of section cuts the aorta (A), the superior mesenteric artery (Ams), the left renal artery (Ars), the left renal vein (Vrs), and the splenic vein (Vl).

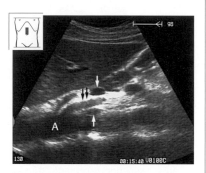

b Ultrasound image corresponding to *a*. Aorta (A), superior mesenteric artery (↓↓), left renal vein (↑), splenic vein (↓).

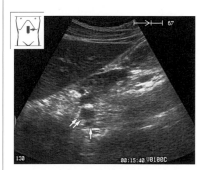

c The transducer was moved to the left. The renal artery (↑) and renal vein (↑↑) appear immediately to the left of the aorta.

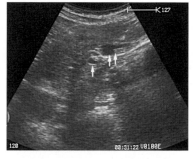

d The transverse was moved farther to the left, demonstrating the renal artery (↑) and renal vein (↑↑) at the hilum.

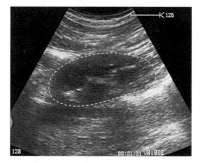

e Scanning farther to the left brings the left kidney (dashed outline) into view.

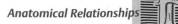
Now return to the starting point over the aorta. Scan to the right in small increments, and watch the aorta disappear. You can now see the right renal artery between the aorta and vena cava. Just above it are the left renal vein and a longitudinal section of the superior mesenteric vein (Fig. 3.**39 a**). Sliding the transducer farther to the right, you will see the vena cava and the right renal artery crossing behind it (Fig. 3.**39 b**). Keep the artery in view and move the transducer farther to the right. The right renal vein will appear, having emerged from the vena cava (Fig. 3.**39 c**). Track the right renal vein and artery to the renal hilum (Fig. 3.**39 d**). The course of the right renal vessels is shown schematically in Fig. 3.**39 e**.

Fig. 3.39 *Demonstrating the right renal vessels in longitudinal section*

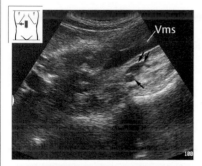

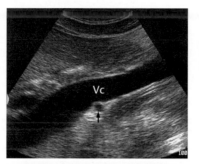

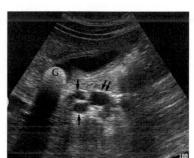

a Longitudinal scan between the aorta and vena cava. You see the right renal artery (↑), left renal vein (↓↓), and superior mesenteric vein (Vms).

b The transducer was moved to the right. You see the vena cava (Vc), which crosses over the right renal artery (↑).

c The transducer was moved farther to the right. You still see the right renal artery, which has split into branches (↑ and ↓), plus the right renal vein (↓↓). A gallstone (G) is noted as an incidental finding.

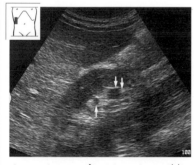

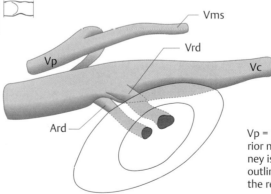

d Renal artery (↑) and renal vein (↓↓) at the hilum.

e Diagram corresponding to image **d**. Note how the right renal vessels (vein and artery) run to and behind the vena cava (Vc), respectively.

Vp = portal vein, Vms = superior mesenteric vein. The kidney is shown in transparent outline so that you can see the renal artery and vein.

37

Iliac vessels

The aorta and vena cava bifurcate just above the promontory into the common iliac arteries and veins, which project on to the abdominal wall at about the level of the umbilicus. After a few centimeters, they divide into the internal and external iliac vessels (Fig. 3.**40**).

Fig. 3.40 Anatomy of the iliac vessels

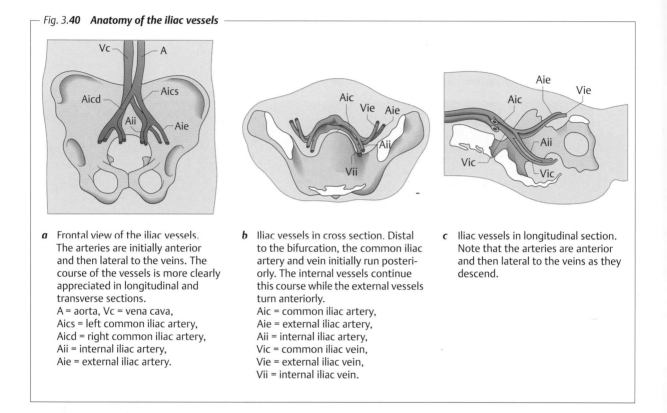

a Frontal view of the iliac vessels. The arteries are initially anterior and then lateral to the veins. The course of the vessels is more clearly appreciated in longitudinal and transverse sections.
A = aorta, Vc = vena cava,
Aics = left common iliac artery,
Aicd = right common iliac artery,
Aii = internal iliac artery,
Aie = external iliac artery.

b Iliac vessels in cross section. Distal to the bifurcation, the common iliac artery and vein initially run posteriorly. The internal vessels continue this course while the external vessels turn anteriorly.
Aic = common iliac artery,
Aie = external iliac artery,
Aii = internal iliac artery,
Vic = common iliac vein,
Vie = external iliac vein,
Vii = internal iliac vein.

c Iliac vessels in longitudinal section. Note that the arteries are anterior and then lateral to the veins as they descend.

The iliac vessels are demonstrated in three sections: a lower abdominal transverse scan (plane 1), a transverse scan through the vessels (plane 2), and a longitudinal scan through the vessels (plane 3) (Fig. 3.**41**).

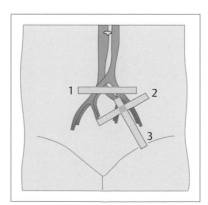

Fig. 3.41 The three scan planes used in examining the iliac vessels.
1 = Lower abdominal transverse scan,
2 = Transverse scan over the vessels,
3 = Longitudinal scan over the vessels.

Demonstrating the iliac vessels in a lower abdominal transverse scan

Place the probe transversely below the umbilicus (plane 1 in Fig. 3.**41**) and scan slightly cephalad to visualize the distal aorta and vena cava in cross section. As you scan slowly downward from there, observe how the two vessels divide (Figs. 3.**42a, b**). As the scan moves lower, the sections of the right and left iliac vessels will move laterally and posteriorly in the field of view (Fig. 3.**42c**). Visualization usually becomes poor at this level due to interposed bowel gas. Return the transducer to its starting position.

Fig. 3.42 Demonstrating the iliac vessels in lower abdominal transverse scans

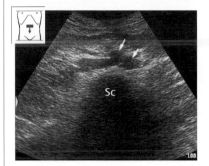

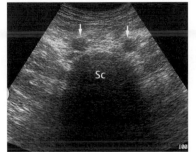

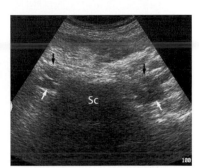

a Section at the level of the aortic bifurcation (↓↓). Sc = spinal column.

b The transducer was moved distally, demonstrating the common iliac arteries (↓).

c As the transducer moves farther distally, the vascular sections move laterally and posteriorly. Common iliac arteries (↓), common iliac veins (↑).

Demonstrating the iliac vessels in transverse section

Rotate the transducer to a plane that is perpendicular to the course of the iliac vessels (plane 2 in Fig. 3.**41**). Track their cross sections distally, gaining an appreciation of the three-dimensional course of the vessels. Identify the artery and vein.

Demonstrating the iliac vessels in longitudinal section

Rotate the transducer to a longitudinal orientation over the iliac vessels (plane 3 in Fig. 3.**41**). Scan across the longitudinal section (Fig. 3.**43a**) and then move the transducer caudad (Fig. 3.**43b**). Identify the origin of the internal iliac artery. Beyond this point, visualization is usually seriously degraded by overlying bowel gas (Fig. 3.**43c**).

*Fig. 3.**43*** *Demonstrating the left iliac vessels in longitudinal section*

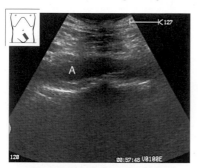

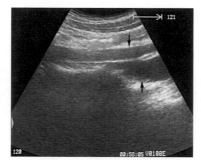

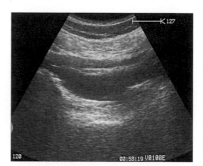

a Longitudinal scan in the area of the bifurcation on the left side. A = aorta.

b The transducer was moved distally along the vessels. Common iliac artery (↓), common iliac vein (↑).

c The transducer was moved farther distally. Visualization at this level is obscured by overlying bowel gas.

Lymph nodes near the retroperitoneal vessels

The intra-abdominal lymph nodes that can be seen with ultrasound are located in close proximity to blood vessels. Thus, the vascular examination should include a routine search for enlarged lymph nodes. Lymph node enlargement may be due to inflammation, metastatic involvement, or malignant lymphoma. Under favorable imaging conditions, a high-resolution scanner can define lymph nodes from 0.5 to 1 cm in size. Lymph nodes 1 cm or more in diameter are considered suspicious.

KEY POINT

Lymph nodes 1 cm or larger are considered suspicious.

Location of lymph nodes

The parietal lymph nodes are distributed along the aorta, vena cava, and iliac vessels. They drain the lower extremities and the organs of the lesser pelvis and retroperitoneum. The visceral lymph nodes drain the gastrointestinal tract, pancreas, liver, and gallbladder. They are located anterior to the iliac vessels and distal aorta, and are distributed along the superior mesenteric artery and vein, the celiac trunk, and the hilar vessels of the liver, spleen, and kidney. Imaging lymph nodes that lie along small vessels can be particularly challenging and requires a meticulous scanning technique in suitably selected cases.

Table 3.**4** reviews the parietal and visceral lymph node groups that are found along abdominal vessels.

Table 3.**4** Parietal and visceral lymph nodes distributed along the abdominal vessels

Parietal	Visceral
Vena cava	Aorta
Aorta	Iliac vessels
Iliac vessels	Inferior mesenteric artery
	Superior mesenteric artery
	Celiac trunk
	Porta hepatis
	Splenic hilum

Ultrasound appearance

There are no well-established criteria for distinguishing between benign and malignant lymph nodes. Different textbooks have offered somewhat different guidelines.

Inflamed lymph nodes tend to be relatively small (< 2 cm), have an oblong shape, and are hypoechoic. Lymph node inflammation in the porta hepatis may be due to acute hepatitis, but inflammatory lymph node changes are also seen in chronic diseases of the liver (Fig. 3.**44**) and biliary tract. The lymph nodes in chronic inflammatory bowel diseases usually remain small.

Metastatic lymph nodes have a plump or rounded shape and tend to show high, nonhomogeneous echogenicity (Figs. 3.**45**, 3.**46**).

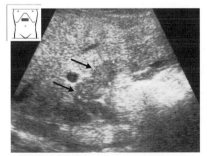

*Fig. 3.**44** Lymph node (→) in the porta hepatis of a patient with chronic hepatitis C.*

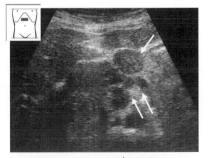

*Fig. 3.**45** Lymph node (↓) at the bifurcation of the celiac trunk (↑↑) in a patient with gastric carcinoma.*

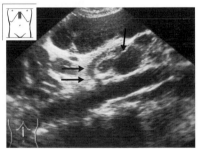

*Fig. 3.**46** Lymph node (↓) on the celiac trunk (→→) in a patient with gastric carcinoma.*

The lymph nodes in patients with malignant lymphoma are large, show uniform low echogenicity, and often have an irregular shape (Figs. 3.**47**, 3.**48**).

When you scan swiftly down major abdominal vessels in transverse sections, enlarged lymph nodes along the vessels will often appear fleetingly in the image as round, hypoechoic masses (Fig. 3.**49**).

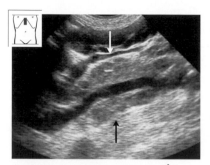 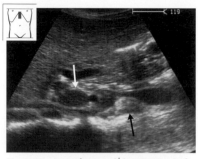 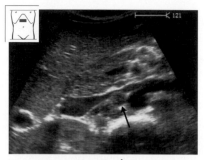

*Fig. 3.**47** Lymphomas posterior (↑) and anterior (↓) to the aorta in a patient with low-grade non-Hodgkin's lymphoma (NHL).*

*Fig. 3.**48** Lymphomas (↓) anterior and posterior to the aorta and vena cava in a patient with malignant NHL.*

*Fig. 3.**49** Lymph node (↑) between the vena cava and aorta.*

Differential diagnosis

Two potential pitfalls in differential diagnosis should be mentioned at this point: the horseshoe kidney and the accessory spleen.

The horseshoe kidney appears as a rounded mass located anterior to the aorta in longitudinal section (p. 202) (Fig. 3.**50**). Even in transverse sections, it can be difficult to trace the anterior mass to the right and left kidneys due to intervening bowel gas.

An accessory spleen cannot be distinguished from a lymph node with absolute certainty. Typically, however, it appears as a homogeneous mass that is isoechoic to the spleen (Fig. 3.**51**).

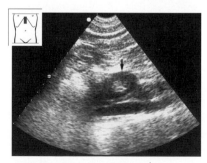 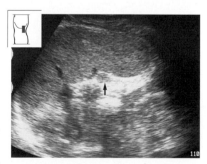

*Fig. 3.**50** Horseshoe kidney (↓),* appearing as an oval mass anterior to the aorta in longitudinal section.

*Fig. 3.**51** Accessory spleen (↑).* Small, spherical accessory spleen of the same echogenicity as the spleen, located on a vessel in the splenic hilum.

4 Liver

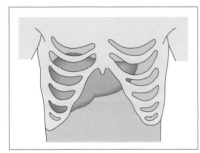

Organ Boundaries

LEARNING GOALS

➤ Locate the liver.
➤ Clearly delineate the liver from its surroundings.
➤ Survey the total liver volume in multiple planes.
➤ Recognize portions of the liver that are difficult to scan.

*Fig. 4.**1** **Approaches for scanning the liver.***

The liver is the dominant organ of the right upper abdomen. It is protected by ribs and is covered mainly by the right costal arch. These simple anatomical facts are widely known, but they have special significance and implications for ultrasound scanning.

1 The liver is so large that cannot be scanned adequately from one approach. A complete examination of the liver requires scanning from multiple angles and directions.

2 The liver cannot be scanned by the shortest route, but only from beneath the costal arch or between the ribs (Fig. 4.**1**). This means that while performing serial scans, you will view many sections of the liver more than once but are apt to miss blind spots if you are not fully familiar with the extent of the organ. Figure 4.**2** illustrates this problem with an analogy.

Locating the liver

*Fig. 4.**2** **Difficulties of liver scanning.*** In this analogy, an observer is looking into a room through three windows. Moving from window to window, he views the center of the room several times and sees corners a total of five times. Even so, he is unable to see the man sitting in one corner of the room.

Barriers to scanning

➤ Ribs
➤ A high diaphragm

Optimizing the scanning conditions

To make the liver more accessible, have the patient raise the right arm above the head to draw the rib cage upward. Place the patient in the supine position and have him or her take a deep breath and hold it to expand the abdomen. One disadvantage of holding the breath is that it is followed by a period of hyperventilation, especially in older patients.

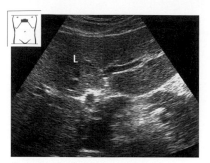

Fig. 4.3   The liver (L) in upper abdominal transverse section.

Organ identification

Start with the transducer placed transversely against the right costal arch, at the level where you would palpate the inferior border of the liver. Mentally picture the liver lying beneath the ribs, and angle the scan upward. Now ask the patient to take a deep breath, expanding the abdomen, and the liver will appear on the screen as a region of homogeneous echo texture. Figure 4.3 illustrates the view of the liver that is acceptable for organ identification.

Imaging the liver in its entirety

Because the liver is so large, it is best to proceed in steps when learning how to scan the entire organ.
1 Learn the outlines of the liver:
   – the inferior border,
   – the superior border,
   – the left border.
2 Survey the liver volume:
   – in longitudinal sections,
   – in subcostal transverse and oblique sections,
   – in intercostal sections.

Outlines of the liver

Defining the inferior border of the liver

The liver tapers inferiorly to a more or less sharp-angled border. This inferior border is easy to demonstrate with ultrasound. Place the transducer longitudinally on the upper abdomen, slightly to the right of the midline. Press the caudal end of the transducer a bit more deeply into the abdominal wall than the cranial end, so that the scan is directed slightly upward. This should bring the sharp inferior hepatic border into view (Fig. 4.4 a).

Now slide the transducer to the left, keeping it in a longitudinal plane while following the line of the costal arch as closely as possible. Also, make sure that the inferior border of the liver stays at the right edge of the image. You can do this by varying the pressure on the transducer as needed.

As the transducer moves farther to the left, the cross section of the liver diminishes in size. Its roughly triangular outline becomes progressively smaller and finally disappears. The image is now dominated by a chaotic pattern of highly contrasting light and dark areas with no discernible shape, caused by the gas and liquid contents of the stomach.

Now return to the starting point and scan past it toward the right side. As you track across the abdomen, you will recognize the aorta and then the vena cava. As you scan past the vena cava, the gallbladder can be identified as a "black" structure in the fasted patient. With luck, the right kidney may also be seen. As the transducer moves farther to the right, the angle of the inferior hepatic border becomes increasingly blunted (Fig. 4.4 b, c).

Visualization often becomes poor at this point, especially in obese patients and when there is interposed gas in the right colic flexure. It can be helpful to have the patient breathe in deeply and inflate the abdomen.

The series of images in Fig. 4.4 were selected to illustrate good scanning conditions. You should keep this in mind if you do not achieve the desired result right away. Figure 4.5 shows the appearance of a liver that is difficult to scan. This scan corresponds to the section in Fig. 4.4 b.

TIPS

To define the inferior border of the liver in longitudinal sections, press the caudal end of the transducer a little more firmly into the abdominal wall than the cranial end.

By varying the pressure on the transducer, you can keep the inferior border of the liver at the right edge of the image.

If there is intervening gas in the right colic flexure, have the patient take a deep breath to expand the abdomen.

Fig. 4.**4**   *Demonstrating the inferior border of the liver*

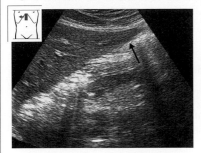

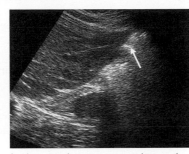

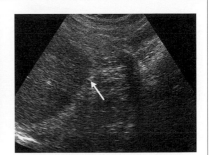

a Scan of the left hepatic lobe, with the transducer placed approximately in the midline. Note the sharp angle of the inferior border (↑).

b The transducer was moved toward the right side, approximately to the midclavicular line. The inferior border appears less sharp (↑).

c The transducer was moved farther to the right. Now the inferior border cannot be clearly defined. The angle is relatively blunt (↑).

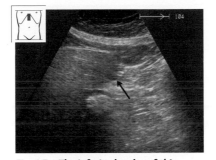

Fig. 4.**5**   *The inferior border of this liver (↑) is difficult to scan.*

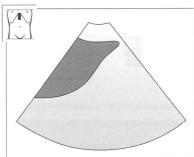

Fig. 4.**6**   *Shape of the inferior border.* Note that the posterior surface of the liver is concave below (toward the inferior border) and convex above.

After you have scanned across the inferior border of the liver once for orientation, make a second pass while giving attention to details. You have already seen that the inferior border has an approximately triangular shape in the ultrasound image. The anterior surface of the liver, which lies against the abdominal wall, is flat and smooth. The posterior surface is slightly concave in its lower portion and becomes slightly convex superiorly (Fig. 4.**6**). The angle between the anterior and posterior surfaces is 30–45° on the left side and 45–70° on the right side (Fig. 4.**7**). The posterior surface has several concavities that interrupt its triangular shape: the porta hepatis and the impressions from the gallbladder and right kidney.

Fig. 4.**7**   *Angle of the inferior border*

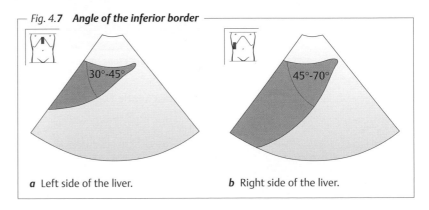

30°–45°   45°–70°

a Left side of the liver.

b Right side of the liver.

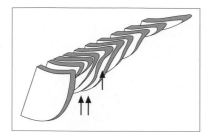

Fig. 4.8 **Longitudinal serial scans of the inferior border.** The posterior surface of the liver bears impressions from the gallbladder (↑) and right kidney (↑↑).

Figure **4.8** illustrates a series of longitudinal sections of the inferior hepatic border obtained by scanning across the liver from left to right. Notice the changes in the liver outline caused by the gallbladder and kidney.

Abnormalities and variants of the inferior border

Fatty liver. Besides increased echogenicity (see p. 53 ff.), fatty infiltration of the liver leads to rounding and broadening of the inferior border (Figs. **4.9**, **4.10**).

Cirrhosis of the liver. The normal liver presents a smooth inferior surface contour. With cirrhosis, regenerative nodules in the liver produce a lobulated contour (Fig. **4.11**).

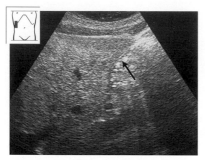

Fig. 4.9 **Fatty liver.** The angle between the anterior and posterior surfaces of the liver is broadened (↑).

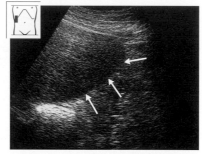

Fig. 4.10 **Fatty liver.** Note the rounding of the inferior border (↑↑↑).

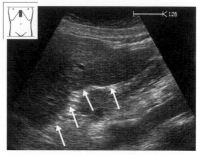

Fig. 4.11 **Alcoholic cirrhosis of the liver.** The inferior surface of the liver has a nodular appearance (↑↑↑).

Riedel's lobe. Riedel's lobe is a tongue-like inferior projection of the right lobe that extends well past the lower pole of the kidney (Fig. **4.12**).

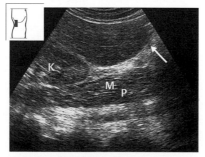

Fig. 4.12 **Riedel's lobe.** A tongue-like projection of the right lobe (↑) extends down past the inferior pole of the kidney. Mp = psoas muscle, N = kidney.

Defining the superior border of the liver

The superior border of the liver is flat on the left side and convex on the right side. The scanning technique is similar to that for the inferior border. Place the transducer longitudinally to the right of the midline just below the costal arch. Angle upward until the superior border of the liver appears on the left side of the screen. Notice the bright echo return from the diaphragm. The pulsating heart can be seen cranially (left side of the image).

Now scan toward the left in parallel longitudinal sections, following the line of the costal arch, until you reach the end of the liver. Then return to the right and continue the scan along the right costal arch (Fig. 4.**13**). You will need to apply firmer transducer pressure in this region in order to scan beneath the ribs at a relatively flat angle.

Fig. 4.13   Demonstrating the superior border of the liver

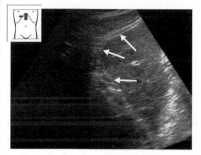 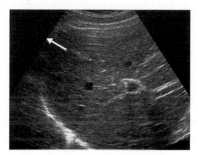 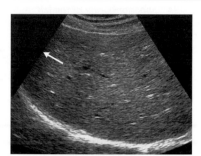

a Superior border of the left lobe (↑↑↑). The transducer was placed approximately in the midline.

b The transducer was moved to the right. Notice that the liver does not transcend the left edge of the image, indicating a complete section (↑).

c The transducer was moved farther to the right. Now the anterior superior portion of the liver is not included in the image (↑). Compare this scan with Fig. 4.**15**.

Repeat the longitudinal pass along the superior border of the liver, this time noticing the shape of the hepatic cross section. The superior border of the liver is flat on the left side. The heart rests upon the diaphragm in this area. The superior surface of the liver forms a right angle with its anterior surface (Fig. 4.**14**). The farther the transducer is moved toward the right, the more convex the surface becomes. At this point you will have to press harder on the transducer and scan beneath the ribs at a relatively steep angle to view the part of the diaphragm that borders the liver. Even so, it is often not possible to define the full cross section of the liver on the left side of the screen, and a portion of the liver will appear cut off (Fig. 4.**15**).

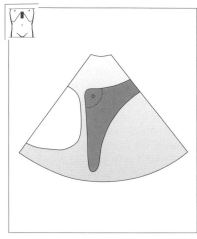

Fig. 4.14 Superior border of the left lobe. Notice the right angle formed by the anterior and diaphragmatic surfaces of the liver.

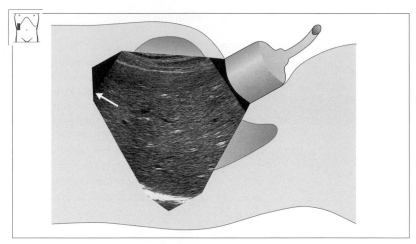

Fig. 4.15 Superior border of the right lobe. Notice that the anterior border cannot be adequately defined.

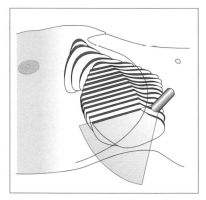

Fig. 4.16 Scanning across the superior border of the liver. Notice that the anterior portions of the right lobe are not visualized.

Try to picture mentally which portion of the liver is not seen. Recall that in a longitudinal scan, the left side of the screen is cranial and the right side is caudal. But as the transducer is angled cephalad, the angle of the scan becomes more horizontal and this rule becomes less valid. With a flat scanning angle, anterior portions of the liver are displayed on the left side of the screen. For our purposes, this means that the hidden, "truncated" portion of the liver cross section is anterior and superior. This blind spot is shown schematically in Fig. 4.**16**.

Defining the left border of the liver

The left border of the liver was already seen in the longitudinal sections of the superior and inferior borders. Now you will also scan down the left border in transverse sections. Place the transducer in a transverse or slightly oblique position along the costal arch, a little to the left of the midline. Scan up toward the liver beneath the costal arch, angling the probe upward until you see the pulsating heart. Scan at a very steep angle so that the left border of the liver is just visible on the screen. Now scan down the left border by angling the transducer. Notice how the shape of the liver section changes as the scan moves downward, changing from trapezoidal above (Fig. 4.**17a**) to triangular below (Fig. 4.**17b**, **c**).

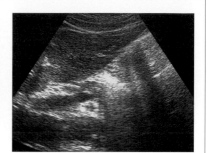

Fig. 4.**17**   *Scanning down the left border of the liver*

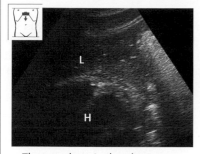 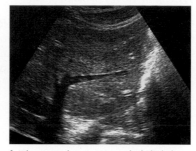 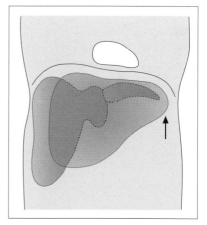

a The transducer is placed transversely on the costal arch and angled sharply upward into the upper abdomen to obtain a tangential, almost coronal scan. Sections of the liver (L) and heart (H) can be seen.

b The transducer was angled slightly downward. The heart is no longer visualized.

c The transducer angle was lowered farther. Now the scan plane passes almost horizontally through the upper abdomen.

This phenomenon is somewhat difficult to understand, since the left border of the liver does not have a trapezoidal shape even in a high transverse section. But it can be explained by the position of the transducer. Angling up into the liver produces a very tangential scan that does not portray a true upper abdominal transverse section; instead, it produces an almost coronal section. Figures 4.**18** and 4.**19** explain this phenomenon.

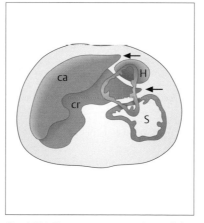

Fig. 4.**18**   *Two transverse sections of the left border of the liver: caudal (ca) in front and cranial (cr) behind.* In the cranial section, the stomach (S) and heart (H) are displayed along with the liver. Notice that the left border of the liver forms a sharp angle (←) in both sections.

Fig. 4.**19**   *Two coronal sections of the liver: anterior in front and posterior behind.* Notice the blunted appearance of the hepatic border (↑) in the anterior coronal section.

In summary, the two figures show the following: As you scan down the hepatic left border, the liver is first imaged in anterior coronal sections. The section of the liver has a trapezoidal shape at this level. But as the scan is angled lower, the more posterior and inferior portions of the liver are displayed in transverse planes. These sections show a more triangular, sharply angled border.

49

Systematic survey of liver volume

Now that you have acquired a feel for the boundaries of the liver, you will learn how to survey the total liver volume. You should get to know the liver in three dimensions. Recall that three basic scanning approaches are available: longitudinal (Fig. 4.**20a**), subcostal transverse or oblique (Fig. 4.**20b**), and intercostal (Fig. 4.**20c**).

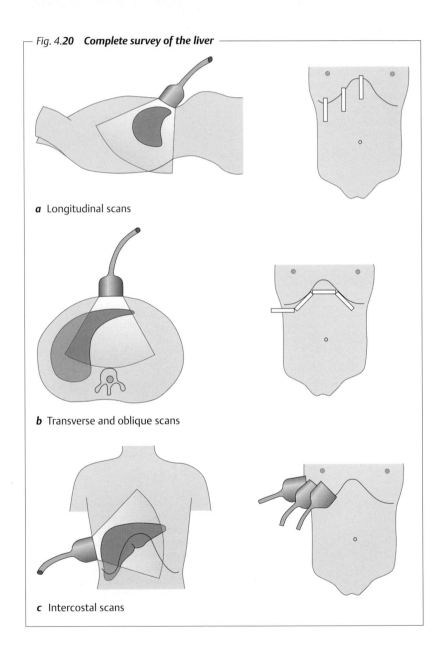

*Fig. 4.**20**   **Complete survey of the liver***

a Longitudinal scans

b Transverse and oblique scans

c Intercostal scans

Scanning across the liver in longitudinal sections

The first step in defining the inferior and superior borders of the liver has already been taken: scanning across the organ in longitudinal sections, making one pass over the inferior portions and another over the superior portions (Figs. 4.**4** and 4.**13**). Remember that the superior portions of the right lobe are a "blind spot" in the longitudinal liver survey.

Scanning the liver in subcostal oblique and transverse sections

Whereas the longitudinal liver sonography is done in parallel planes, subcostal scans are swept through the liver in a fan-shaped pattern. Four or five of these sweeps are necessary for a complete survey. The scans proceed from left to right, following the costal margins.

Place the transducer in the epigastrium to the left of the midline, as for imaging the left hepatic border, and sweep the scan in a fan-shaped pattern as you did before (Fig. 4.**21**).

Fig. 4.**21** *Scanning the liver in transverse sections: center of the liver*

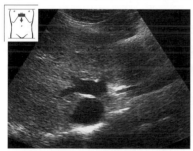
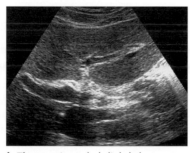
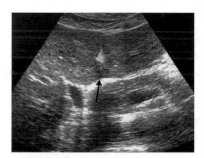

a The transducer is placed transversely at the center of the upper abdomen and angled obliquely upward.

b The scan is angled slightly lower.

c The scan angle is lowered farther. The cross section of the liver has become relatively narrow (↑). The scan plane is perpendicular to the abdominal wall.

You can also hold the transducer in a slightly oblique position, parallel to the costal margin. The liver can be scanned in the same fashion from other probe placements (Figs. 4.**20 b**, 4.**22**).

Fig. 4.**22** *Scanning the liver in transverse sections: right lobe*

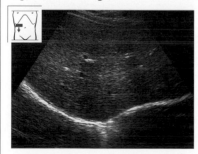
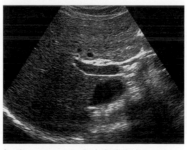
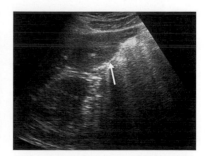

a The transducer is placed transversely to the right of the midline, with the scan angled obliquely upward.

b The scan is angled slightly lower.

c The scan angle is lowered farther. The cross section of the liver has become relatively narrow (↑). The scan plane is perpendicular to the abdominal wall.

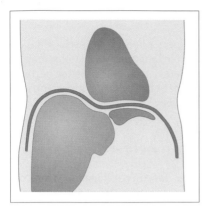

Fig. 4.23   Relative positions of the left and right hemidiaphragms.

Repeat this pass and notice that the dome of the left lobe can be seen relatively clearly while that of the right lobe is indistinct, especially anteriorly. The left lobe is easier to visualize because it is being scanned through the epigastrium and because the left hemidiaphragm is lower than the right (Fig. 4.**23**).

Scanning the liver in intercostal sections

The third scanning approach to the liver is the one through the intercostal spaces. Picture the course of the ribs in the lateral and anterior portions of the costal arch. Reinforce this by palpating the subject's ribs. The scan planes are directed between adjacent ribs.

Intercostal scans are part of every upper abdominal ultrasound examination. To help you learn this approach, we shall describe it here in considerably more detail than is usually done.

Intercostal scanning follows a three-step routine:
1   Scan through the liver in a fan-shaped pattern.
2   Slide the transducer along the intercostal space and repeat step 1.
3   Move the transducer to the next intercostal space and repeat steps 1 and 2.

Place the transducer in a laterally and somewhat posteriorly situated intercostal space (ICS). Take care to direct the scan plane parallel to the ribs. Define the liver, and angle the transducer to sector the scan through the accessible liver segment (Fig. 4.**24**). Then slide the transducer cranially and caudally within the same ICS and repeat the sectoring maneuver. Next, move the transducer to the medially adjacent ICS and carefully repeat the process. Stick to this routine in the beginning, even if it seems somewhat tedious.

When you have done this exercise, picture the portions of the liver that you have scanned. The areas located close to the chest wall and transducer are the areas that are poorly visualized in subcostal longitudinal, oblique, and transverse scans. The posterior portions of the liver located farther from the transducer were already visualized through the subcostal approach.

*Fig. 4.**24**   Scanning the liver in intercostal sections*

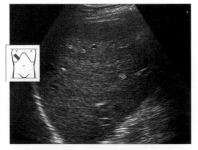

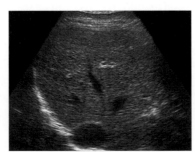

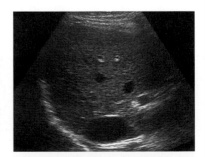

a The transducer is placed in a laterally situated ICS. The scan is angled steeply upward.

b The transducer is angled slightly lower.

c The transducer is angled still lower. The scan plane is now perpendicular to the body surface.

Organ Details

> **LEARNING GOALS**
>
> ➤ Evaluate the shape of the liver.
> ➤ Determine the size of the liver.
> ➤ Evaluate the parenchymal pattern.
> ➤ Evaluate the veins, portal vessels, ligaments, and fissures within the parenchyma.

Shape

The outlines of the liver were covered in the previous section. Deviations from normal findings include an increased angle at the anterior border of the liver, blunting of the hepatic border, and irregularities in the normally smooth liver contour (see p. 46).

Size

The craniocaudal extent of the right lobe is generally said to be 12–13 cm at the midclavicular line, although the normal liver is quite variable in size.

Parenchymal pattern

The parenchyma of the liver shows a moderately dense, homogeneous echo pattern. The renal parenchyma, which is slightly hypoechoic to the liver, is used as a reference for evaluating hepatic echogenicity (Fig. 4.**25**).

Abnormalities of the liver parenchyma: diffuse changes

Fatty liver. One of the most common findings at ultrasound is increased echogenicity of the liver due to fatty infiltration. This may be caused by overeating, alcohol abuse, hepatitis, diabetes mellitus, disorders of lipid metabolism, or medications. The fatty liver is characterized by increased echogenicity relative to the renal parenchyma (Fig. 4.**26**) and distal sound attenuation (Fig. 4.**27**). Scans may also show rounding of the inferior hepatic border (see p. 46) and narrowing of the hepatic veins (see p. 61).

Bright portal vessels. Occasionally, cross sections of the portal vessels appear as very bright echoes in a completely healthy liver (Fig. 4.**28**).

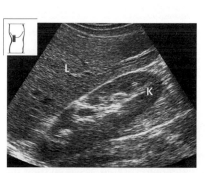

*Fig. 4.**25** **Normal echo pattern of the liver.** The parenchyma of the liver (L) has approximately the same echogenicity as the renal parenchyma (K).

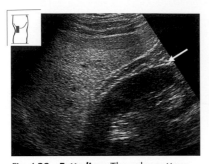

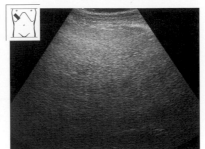

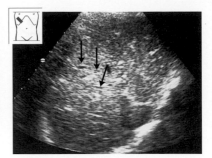

Fig. 4.26 **Fatty liver.** The echo pattern of the liver is markedly denser than that of the kidney. Note also the conspicuous perirenal fat (←).

Fig. 4.27 **Fatty liver.** The sound is markedly attenuated in the deep part of the field. Vessels are poorly delineated. Hypertriglyceridemia.

Fig. 4.28 **Normal variant.** Strongly echogenic portal vessels (↓↓↓).

Cirrhosis of the liver. Cirrhosis of the liver is characterized by an unsettled parenchymal pattern with fine or coarse granularity (see also p. 61) (Fig. 4.**29**).

Hepatic metastases. Extensive metastatic deposits can create a very nonhomogeneous pattern that involves the entire liver and may be difficult to interpret (Fig. 4.**30**).

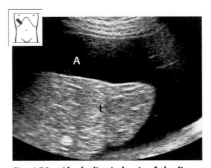

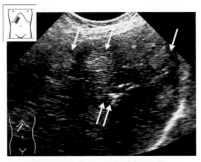

Fig. 4.29 **Alcoholic cirrhosis of the liver.** The echo pattern shows increased density. The liver (L) is small and surrounded by ascites (A).

Fig. 4.30 **Liver permeated by metastases.** Ultrasound shows a very nonhomogeneous pattern, consisting of echogenic areas (↓) and calcifications (↑↑) in a very unsettled parenchyma.

Abnormalities of the liver parenchyma: circumscribed changes

Circumscribed changes in the liver parenchyma are often challenging for the sonographer. Many findings can be adequately interpreted based on their ultrasound features, whereas others will require additional studies. When a circumscribed change is discovered in the liver, the examiner should systematically evaluate the following features:

➤ *Echogenicity:* echo-free, hypoechoic, isoechoic, echogenic, highly echogenic, posterior enhancement, shadowing.
➤ *Shape:* round, oval, scalloped, irregular, triangular, polygonal.
➤ *Margins:* sharp, ill-defined.
➤ *Size:* measured in at least two dimensions.
➤ *Internal structure:* homogeneous/nonhomogeneous, hypoechoic/hyperechoic border, hypoechoic/hyperechoic center.
➤ *Number:* solitary, multiple, numerous.
➤ *Location:* intrahepatic (right, left, segment), perivascular.
➤ *Relation to surroundings:* expansile, infiltrating.

Echo-free lesions

Solitary nonparasitic cysts. These lesions are clearly visible when approximately 5 mm or larger. Solitary hepatic cysts, usually congenital, are found in up to 4% of the adult population. They are characterized by a round or oval shape, smooth margins, a thin wall, no internal echoes, posterior acoustic enhancement, and lateral edge shadows (Figs. 4.**31**, 4.**32**). They can be diagnosed sonographically. Multiple cysts are much less common (Fig. 4.**33**).

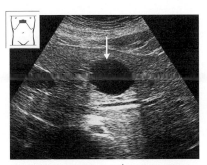

Fig. 4.31 Hepatic cyst (↓). Notice the smooth, round margins, the echo-free cyst wall, the posterior acoustic enhancement, and the lateral edge shadows.

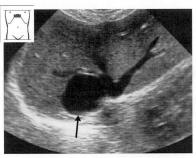

Fig. 4.32 Solitary hepatic cyst with compression of the right hepatic vein (↑).

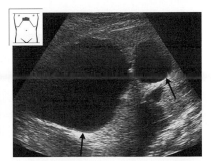

Fig. 4.33 Multiple hepatic cysts (↑↑), one of which is 8 cm in diameter.

Table 4.**1**   Echo-free hepatic lesions

Nonparasitic hepatic cyst
Hydatid cyst
Concentric biliary tract dilatation (Caroli syndrome)
Liver abscess

Cystic liver. Hereditary cystic liver disease is characterized by cysts of varying size that permeate the liver (Figs. 4.**34**, 4.**35**).

Parasitic cysts. The cysts caused by infection with *Echinococcus granulosus* are characterized by an echogenic wall. It is common to find septations and adjacent daughter cysts (Fig. 4.**36**).

The differential diagnosis of echo-free hepatic lesions is reviewed in Table 4.**1**.

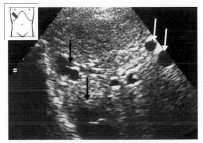

Fig. 4.34 Multiple cysts of varying size (↓), numbering more than 20 in all.

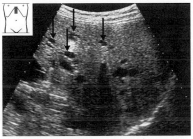

Fig. 4.35 Multiple cysts (↓).

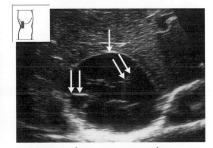

Fig. 4.36 Echinococcus granulosus infection. Large, loculated cyst (↓) with conspicuous septa (↓↓). Note the relatively bright wall echoes.

Metastasis
Adenoma
Focal nodular hyperplasia
Atypical hemangioma
Hepatocellular carcinoma
Abscess
Focal sparing from fatty infiltration
Hematoma

Hypoechoic lesions

Hypoechoic lesions in the liver can be difficult to interpret in some cases. Lesions with a round or oval shape are always suspicious for metastasis. Other causes are listed in Table 4.**2**.

Metastases (Figs. 4.**37** – 4.**42**). Hepatic metastases may appear as hypoechoic lesions (Figs. 4.**37**, 4.**38**), or they may be isoechoic or hyperechoic. They may be relatively homogeneous, especially when small, but typically appear as a target lesion with a hypoechoic rim (Figs. 4.**40**, 4.**41**).

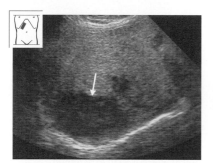

*Fig. 4.**37*** **Hepatic metastases from breast carcinoma (↓).** Rounded, hypoechoic, homogeneous metastasis without a halo.

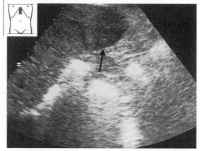

*Fig. 4.**38*** **Hepatic metastasis from colon carcinoma (↑).** Rounded, hypoechoic, predominantly homogeneous metastasis without a halo.

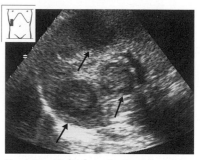

*Fig. 4.**39*** **Multiple metastases from bronchial carcinoma (↑).**

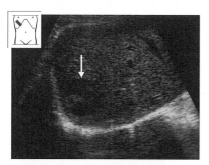

*Fig. 4.**40*** **Hepatic metastasis from colon carcinoma (↓),** appearing as a target lesion with a large, hypoechoic halo.

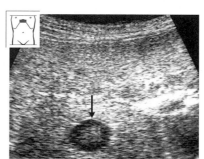

*Fig. 4.**41*** **Hepatic metastasis from uterine carcinoma (↓),** appearing as a target lesion with a somewhat narrow, hypoechoic rim.

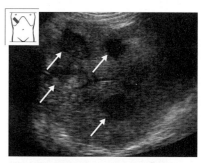

*Fig. 4.**42*** **Hepatic metastases from an unknown primary tumor (↑).** Multiple metastases of varying echogenicity.

Adenoma (Fig. 4.**43**). Adenomas of the liver are rare lesions that sometimes appear as rounded, hypoechoic, or isoechoic masses. But often they are difficult to delineate. They cannot be positively distinguished from metastases or hepatocellular carcinoma based on ultrasound criteria alone. Adenomas are classified as a precancerous lesion.

Focal nodular hyperplasia (FNH) (Fig. 4.**44**). FNH is a hypoechoic or sometimes isoechoic mass that is often indistinguishable sonographically from an adenoma or atypical hemangioma.

Atypical hemangioma. Whereas a typical hemangioma is echogenic, atypical hemangiomas may have a hypoechoic, nonhomogeneous appearance.

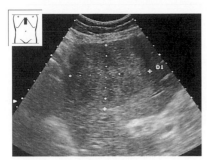

Fig. 4.**43**   **Hepatic adenoma.**

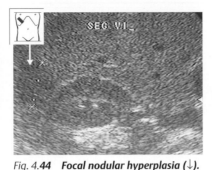

Fig. 4.**44**   **Focal nodular hyperplasia (↓).**

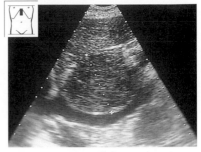

Fig. 4.**45**   **Hepatocellular carcinoma.**

Hepatocellular carcinoma (HCC) (Fig. 4.**45**). Hepatocellular carcinoma is the most common of the primary hepatic malignancies (hepatocellular, cholangiocellular, and mixed). It is found predominantly in cirrhotic livers, appearing as a hypoechoic or sometimes hyperechoic, nonhomogeneous mass. HCC may be solitary or multifocal.

Abscess (Fig. 4.**46**). Abscesses can have a variety of sonographic features, appearing as hypoechoic, nonhomogeneous, or hyperechoic rounded lesions with ill-defined margins.

Focal sparing (Figs. 4.**47**, 4.**48**). This refers to one or more areas of normal liver parenchyma that have been spared by the process of fatty infiltration. Usually they have a triangular or oval shape and are often located near the gallbladder.

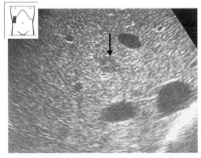

Fig. 4.**46**   **Candida abscess in a patient with HIV infection (↓).**

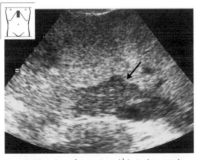

Fig. 4.**47**   **Focal sparing (↓).** Polygonal-shaped area at the inferior border of the liver has been spared from fatty infiltration.

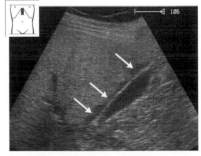

Fig. 4.**48**   **Focal sparing (→).** Very narrow spared area in fatty infiltration, located next to the gallbladder bed.

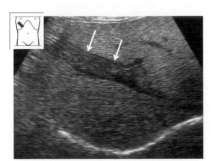

Fig. 4.**49**   **Intrahepatic hematoma (↓).**

Hematoma (Fig. 4.**49**). Hematomas appear as irregular, hypoechoic areas in the liver tissue.

Table 4.**3** Isoechoic hepatic lesions

Focal nodular hyperplasia

Hepatocellular carcinoma

Metastasis

Hemangioma

Isoechoic lesions

Lesions that are isoechoic to the liver parenchyma can be detected by changes in their surroundings (mass effect, halo) or structural differences (Figs. 4.**50**, 4.**51**). They are listed in Table 4.**3**.

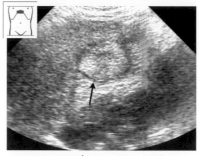

Fig. 4.**50**   **HCC (↑).** Though isoechoic to the surrounding liver tissue, the lesion is clearly delineated by a narrow, hypoechoic rim.

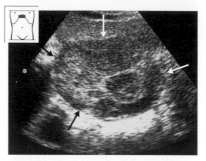

Fig. 4.**51**   **Cavernous hemangioma (→↓←).** Scan shows an approximately isoechoic, somewhat nonhomogeneous, rounded mass at the inferior border of the liver. A hemorrhagic area is visible within the mass.

Table 4.**4** Hyperechoic, non-shadowing hepatic lesions

Metastasis

Hemangioma

Focal nodular hyperplasia

Hepatocellular carcinoma

Focal sparing from fatty infiltration

Ligamentum teres

Hyperechoic, non-shadowing lesions

Hyperechoic, non-shadowing lesions of the liver are listed in Table 4.**4**.

Hemangioma (Figs. 4.**52** – 4.**54**). Hemangiomas are occasionally detected incidentally in the liver. Most of these lesions are very echogenic and have sharp margins without a hypoechoic rim. Generally they have a rounded shape, but irregular forms are also seen. They may be solitary or multiple and are usually smaller than 2 cm. A feeding vessel can often be identified.

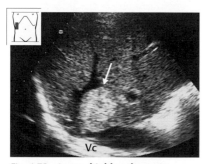

Fig. 4.**52**   **Large, highly echogenic hemangioma compressing the hepatic vein (↓).** Vc = vena cava.

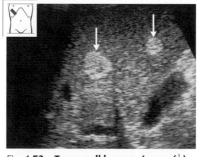

Fig. 4.**53**   **Two small hemangiomas (↓).** The larger of the two lesions has a hypoechoic center.

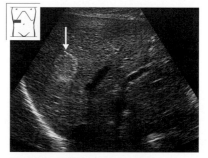

Fig. 4.**54**   **Relatively hypoechoic hemangioma (↓).**

HCC, metastases (Figs. 4.55 – 4.57), and FNH can occasionally appear more echogenic than their surroundings.

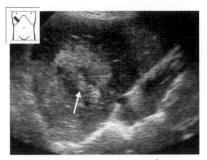

Fig. 4.55 Hepatic metastases (↑). Hyperechoic, relatively homogeneous, irregularly shaped metastases from colon carcinoma in the right lobe of the liver.

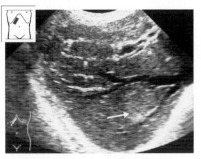

Fig. 4.56 Hepatic metastases (→). Hyperechoic metastases compressing the hepatic vein.

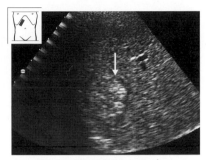

Fig. 4.57 Hepatic metastases (↓). Nonhomogeneous mass containing some high-level echoes, located at the superior border of the liver, in a patient with colon carcinoma.

Table 4.5 Highly echogenic hepatic lesions

Simple calcification
Hemangioma
Metastasis
Air in the bile ducts
Calcified abscess
E. multilocularis

Highly echogenic hepatic lesions that cast an acoustic shadow

These lesions are reviewed in Table 4.5.

Simple calcifications. Simple calcifications are occasionally found in the liver with no apparent cause (Fig. 4.58). Possible causes include trauma and prior infections (Fig. 4.59).

Hemangiomas (Fig. 4.60) and **metastases** (Fig. 4.61). Both types of lesion may contain calcifications.

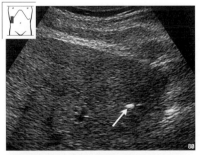

Fig. 4.58 Simple calcification of unknown cause (↑).

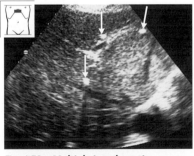

Fig. 4.59 Multiple intrahepatic calcifications in a patient with a prior history of tuberculosis (↓).

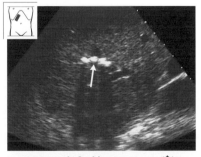

Fig. 4.60 Calcified hemangioma (↑).

Ligamentum teres. The ligamentum teres may be so echogenic in cross section that it casts a posterior acoustic shadow (Fig. 4.**62**).

Air in the bile ducts. Air in the bile ducts typically produces a comet-tail artifact due to the high impedance mismatch (Fig. 4.**63**). This condition can have numerous causes including a previous papillotomy, a stent in the bile duct, a biliary–enteric anastomosis, and cholangitis.

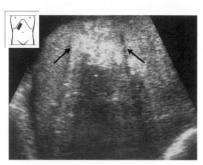

Fig. 4.61   Calcified metastasis (↑). Colon carcinoma.

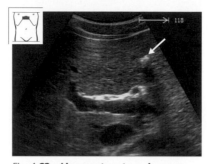

Fig. 4.62   Ligamentum teres in cross section (↓), with an associated acoustic shadow.

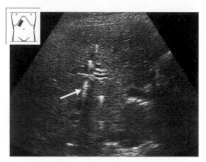

Fig. 4.63   Air in the bile ducts. Comet-tail artifacts (→) are a typical finding.

Vessels of the liver

The portal vein, bile ducts, and hepatic artery follow approximately the same course (Glisson's triad). They are easily identified in the hilum (see p. 96 ff.). The intrahepatic portal vessels are easy to distinguish by their bright wall echoes (Fig. 4.**64**). Generally the bile ducts can be identified near the hilum but not in the periphery, assuming they are not obstructed (Figs. 4.**65**, 4.**66**). The branches of the hepatic artery cannot be visualized within the liver.

   The hepatic veins are clearly identifiable by their direct, gently curving course toward the vena cava and their low-level wall echoes (Fig. 4.**64**). The hepatic veins change their caliber with respiration. They have a maximum diameter of 5 mm before terminating at the vena cava.

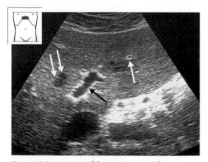

Fig. 4.64   Normal hepatic vessels. Portal vessels (↑) show relatively bright wall echoes, while hepatic veins (↓↓) have less reflective walls.

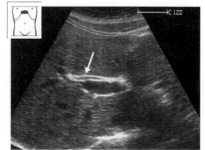

Fig. 4.65   Bile duct. Scan clearly demonstrates an intrahepatic bile duct (↓) located anterior to the right portal vein branch.

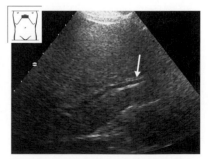

Fig. 4.66   Very fine, normal-appearing bile duct (↓), still visible relatively far into the periphery of the liver.

Abnormalities of the hepatic veins, portal vein branches, and bile ducts

Dilatation of the hepatic veins. Right-sided heart failure (Fig. 4.**67**) leads to the features of a congested liver with hepatomegaly and dilatation of the hepatic veins, whose calibers no longer vary with respiration.

Narrowing of the hepatic veins. Cirrhosis of the liver leads to narrowing and caliber irregularities of the hepatic veins (Fig. 4.**68**).

Portal vein cutoff. Narrowing of the portal vein branches in a cirrhotic liver creates a "truncated" appearance of the portal trunk (Fig. 4.**69**).

The vascular and bile-duct changes that are seen in hepatic cirrhosis are listed in Table 4.**6** along with other sonographic findings that occur in the disease.

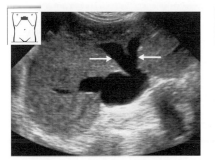

Fig. 4.67 Hepatic venous congestion in a patient with right heart failure (→←).

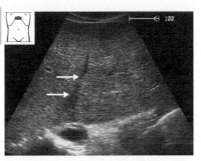

Fig. 4.68 Narrowing and caliber irregularities (→) of the hepatic veins in a cirrhotic liver.

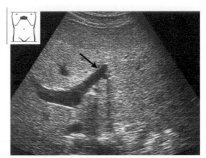

Fig. 4.69 Nonvisualization of the portal vein branches in a cirrhotic liver (→).

Table 4.**6** Summary of the sonographic findings in hepatic cirrhosis

Criterion	Description
Liver size	– Increased in 50% of cases – Decreased in advanced stages – Enlargement of the left lobe, especially the caudate lobe (Fig. 4.**81**)
Liver shape	– Plump, biconvex (Figs. 4.**10**, 4.**29**) – Rounded inferior border (Fig. 4.**10**) – Border angle > 45° (Fig. 4.**9**)
Outlines of liver	– Wavy – Fine or coarse nodularity (Fig. 4.**11**) – Indentations (Fig. 4.**11**)
Structure of liver	– Irregular, hyperechoic, speckled (Fig. 4.**29**) – Posterior acoustic shadowing
Consistency of liver tissue	– Loss of elasticity
Hepatic veins	– Rarefied – Caliber variations (Fig. 4.**68**) – Branching angle > 45°
Portal vein	– Rarefied side branches (Fig. 4.**69**)
Portal hypertension	– Portal vein > 1.5 cm (Fig. 5.**12**) – Cavernous transformation (Fig. 5.**14**) – Splenic vein poorly compressible – Splenic varices – Recanalized umbilical vein (Cruveilhier-von Baumgarten syndrome [Fig. 4.**76 d**])
Gallbladder	– Thickened wall (Fig. 6.**31**) – Increased incidence of stones (Fig. 6.**32**)
Splenomegaly	– Increased incidence
Ascites	– Often present in advanced stages (Figs. 4.**29**, 4.**113 c**).

Dilated bile ducts. Obstructions of the bile ducts lead to a dilatation that is visible with ultrasound (Figs. 4.**70**, 4.**71**). The obstruction may be caused by stones, neoplasia, or inflammatory changes.

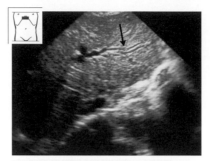

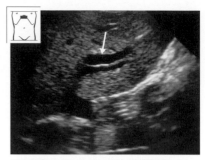

Fig. 4.**70** *Dilated bile ducts, clearly visible in the periphery of the liver (↓).* The "double barrel shotgun" sign.

Fig. 4.**71** *Markedly dilated bile duct (↓) anterior to the portal vein branch.*

Division of the liver into lobes, segments, and subsegments

The sonographically detectable landmarks by which the lobar and segmental boundaries in the liver are identified are ligaments, fissures, hepatic veins, portal vein branches, and certain extrahepatic structures.

The liver is traditionally divided into a left and right lobe based on surface anatomy. This division does not satisfy surgical and functional requirements, however. The functional subdivision of the liver is based on the distribution of intrahepatic vascular structures: The large hepatic veins take an intersegmental course, while the portal vein branches, bile ducts, and hepatic arteries project to the center of the segments. From a functional standpoint, this forms the basis for a lobation scheme of the liver that differs from the classic anatomical scheme.

The major difference between these schemes lies in whether the quadrate lobe and caudate lobe, visible inferior and superiorly when the liver is viewed from behind, are assigned to the right or left lobe. Anatomically, both lobes are considered to belong to the right lobe. Functionally, however, the quadrate lobe belongs to the left lobe while the caudate lobe is considered a separate unit.

The sonographic identification of these four major divisions of the liver — the left lobe (anatomical), caudate lobe, quadrate lobe, and right lobe — and the structures that define their boundaries will be explored below.

It is not easy to recognize the subdivisions of the liver with ultrasound. You should take your time in learning this section of the book and return to it as needed. We suggest that, initially, you devote one hour of concentrated study to this topic, so that you will not become discouraged. You will probably have to review this chapter several times.

First, take a look at a frontal view of the liver as it is pictured in most textbooks of anatomy and ultrasound (Fig. 4.**72**). Notice that the falciform ligament and the externally visible part of the ligamentum teres divide the liver into a right and left lobe. The falciform ligament is attached to the surface of the liver and anchors it to the abdominal wall. It does not extend appreciably into the liver substance and is not visualized with ultrasound. Consequently, it does not help the sonographer in differentiating the right and left lobes. The

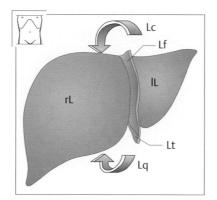

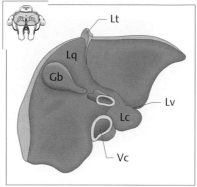

Fig. 4.72   Anterior view of the liver.
The falciform ligament (Lf) divides the liver anatomically into right and left lobes.
Lt = ligamentum teres,
Lc = caudate lobe,
Lq = quadrate lobe,
lL = left lobe,
rL = right lobe.

Fig. 4.73   Upper abdominal transverse scan of the liver. Notice that the ligamentum teres (Lt) marks the boundary of the left lobe. The quadrate lobe (Lq) lies between the ligamentum teres and the gallbladder (Gb). The ligamentum venosum (Lv) separates the caudate lobe (Lc) from the left lobe. The caudate lobe lies between the ligamentum venosum and vena cava (Vc).

ligamentum teres can be seen below the hepatic border in this view. It passes into the liver (this cannot be seen in the diagram) and provides a very useful sonographic landmark.

The sonographic view of the liver in the upper abdominal transverse scan (Fig. 4.**73**) is different from the usual frontal view. It is unfamiliar because the liver is rotated 90º and viewed from below. Take a few minutes to study these illustrations.

Ligamentum teres and quadrate lobe

Do you remember what this "round ligament" is and how it originates? It is an obliterated vessel that runs from the umbilicus to the portal vein, or more precisely to its left main branch. It is a remnant of the fetal umbilical vein, which carried oxygenated blood to the inferior vena cava. On reaching the liver surface, the ligament takes a fairly straight course into the liver, running posteriorly upward to the left portal vein branch. The ligamentum teres is the anatomical boundary marker between the left lobe and quadrate lobe. It is not a boundary surface, but a line. The actual boundary surface between the left lobe and quadrate lobe is the sagittal plane that the ligamentum teres occupies. The plane of the gallbladder forms the boundary between the quadrate lobe and right lobe.

Locating and scanning the ligamentum teres in transverse sections

The ligamentum teres is best identified in transverse section. Place the probe transversely on the upper abdomen. Center the vena cava and aorta in the image. Then define the inferior border of the liver in the transverse scan. Often you will already recognize the polygonal outline of the highly reflective ligamentum teres. If you do not see the ligament, angle the transducer slightly cephalad and caudad. If necessary, repeat the angling movements after slid-

Fig. 4.74   Defining the ligamentum teres and quadrate lobe in transverse sections

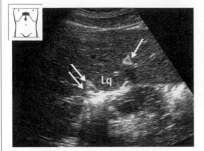

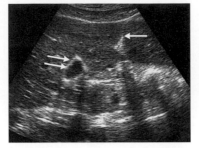

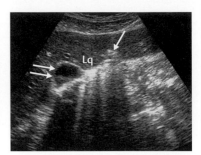

a Angle the transverse scan slightly upward into the liver. You will recognize the triangular outline of the ligamentum teres (↓), the quadrate lobe (Lq), and the start of the gallbladder bed (→→).

b Angling lower, you see the ligamentum teres extending to the hepatic border (←), and the gallbladder comes into view (→→).

c Now the scan plane is perpendicular to the body surface, defining the inferior border of the liver. You see the ligamentum teres (↓), quadrate lobe (Lq), and gallbladder (→→).

d Notice in the diagram that the quadrate lobe (Lq) protrudes between the gallbladder (Gb) and ligamentum teres (Lt) in the transverse section.

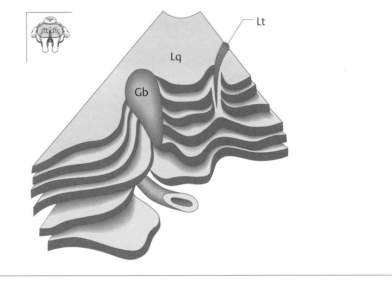

ing the transducer a little to the left or right from the starting position. Figure 4.**74 a** shows the typical ultrasound appearance of the ligament.

Next, angle the transducer downward to trace the cross section of the ligamentum teres in the craniocaudal direction. Notice that as the scan is angled caudad, the polygonal cross section moves anteriorly, i.e., toward the top of the image (Fig. 4.**74 b**). Its cross section at this level becomes larger and less echogenic. Trace the ligamentum teres to the inferior border of the liver (Fig. 4.**74 c**). Then angle the transducer back upward and track the ligament back up to the portal vein. Repeat this pass several times, sweeping the scan briskly, and you will gain a three-dimensional impression of the course of the ligament.

Scanning the quadrate lobe in transverse sections

You have gained a spatial impression of the course of the ligamentum teres. Now turn your attention to the structures located to the right and left of the ligament. Select a view that displays the ligamentum teres at about the center of the liver parenchyma (Fig. 4.**74a**). To the left of the ligament (right in the image) is the left lobe. To the right of the ligamentum teres is the quadrate lobe, which you recall is assigned anatomically to the right lobe and functionally to the left lobe.

Now scan slowly down the ligamentum teres again, as you did before, but this time observe the quadrate lobe. Recognize the prominence of the quadrate lobe and notice the gallbladder appearing at the inferior border of the liver, on the left side of the screen. It marks the right boundary of the quadrate lobe. These relationships are shown schematically in Fig. 4.**74 d**. Take another look at Fig. 4.**73** and relate it to what you have seen in the scans.

Scanning the ligamentum teres and quadrate lobe in longitudinal sections

Next scan the ligamentum teres in longitudinal sections. Place the probe transversely on the upper abdomen again and demonstrate the now-familiar ligament (Fig. 4.**75a**). While watching the screen, rotate the transducer 90°. The ligamentum teres can now be identified as a narrow band (Fig. 4.**75 b, c**).

Fig. 4.**75** *Locating the ligamentum teres in longitudinal section*

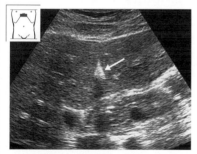

a The ligamentum teres (←) in transverse section.

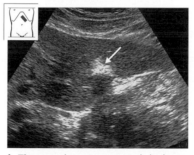

b The transducer was rotated clockwise about 45º. The ligamentum teres appears to lengthen (↓).

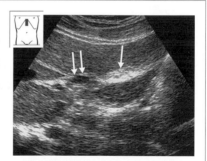

c The transducer was rotated farther to a longitudinal scan. You see the ligamentum teres, which runs from the left portal vein branch (↓↓) to the inferior border of the liver (↓).

Fig. 4.76   Demonstrating the ligamentum teres in longitudinal section

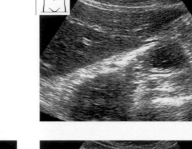

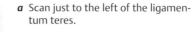

a Scan just to the left of the ligamentum teres.

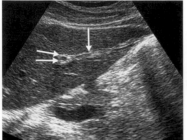

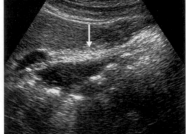

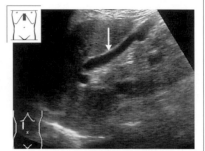

b The transducer was moved a short distance to the right, bringing the ligamentum teres (↓) into view. Note that it runs from the left portal vein branch (→→) to the inferior border of the liver.

c The transducer was moved very slightly to the right. The powerful ligamentum teres (↓) can be recognized.

d Recanalization of the umbilical vein in portal hypertension (↓) (Cruvellhier-von Baumgarten syndrome).

Scan through the ligamentum teres from left to right by angling the transducer slightly. The ability to define the ligament with ultrasound will vary considerably from case to case (Fig. 4.**76**).

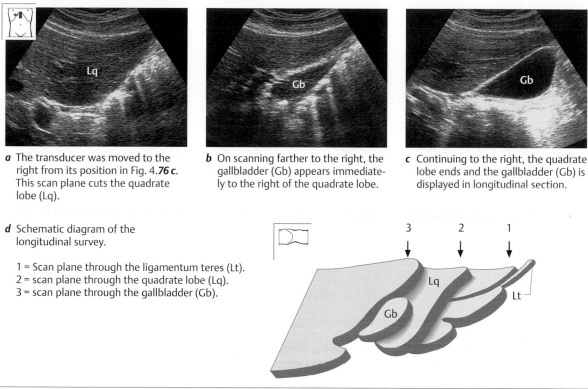

Fig. 4.**77** *Demonstrating the quadrate lobe in longitudinal sections*

a The transducer was moved to the right from its position in Fig. 4.**76 c**. This scan plane cuts the quadrate lobe (Lq).

b On scanning farther to the right, the gallbladder (Gb) appears immediately to the right of the quadrate lobe.

c Continuing to the right, the quadrate lobe ends and the gallbladder (Gb) is displayed in longitudinal section.

d Schematic diagram of the longitudinal survey.

1 = Scan plane through the ligamentum teres (Lt).
2 = scan plane through the quadrate lobe (Lq).
3 = scan plane through the gallbladder (Gb).

Now scan past the ligament toward the right side, proceeding in small steps, until you see the quadrate lobe (Fig. 4.**77 a–c**). It is more difficult to identify in the longitudinal scan than in the transverse scan because the structures bordering it, the gallbladder and ligamentum teres, cannot be displayed simultaneously. This is shown schematically in Fig. 4.**77 d**.

Fissure of the ligamentum venosum, ligamentum venosum, and caudate lobe

You are already familiar with the ligamentum teres and quadrate lobe. We will now familiarize you with two structures that are helpful in delineating the upper portion of the left lobe: the fissure of the ligamentum venosum, in which the ligamentum venosum is lodged, and the caudate lobe. Do not be concerned if you learned these names a while ago and have long forgotten them. You will become reacquainted with them shortly. First, look again at the liver from below, as it presents itself to the sonographer (Fig. 4.**78 a**).

You already know the appearance of the ligamentum teres in this view. In the area where the fissure for the ligamentum teres ends near the porta hepatis, you will find a different ligament that runs upward over the inferior and posterior surface of the liver. It occupies the superficial part of a fissure that curves in front of the caudate lobe and separates it from the left lobe.

The caudate lobe appears as a vaguely sausage-shaped protrusion on the posterosuperior border of the inferior hepatic surface. Notice that the caudate lobe is bounded on the right and posteriorly by the vena cava, and on the left and anteriorly by the fissure of the ligamentum venosum. The ligament that occupies this fissure is the obliterated remnant of the ductus venosus from

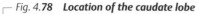

Fig. 4.**78**   *Location of the caudate lobe*

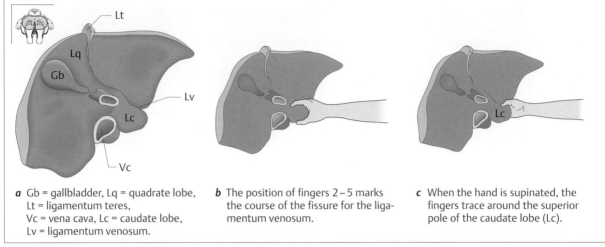

a Gb = gallbladder, Lq = quadrate lobe,
   Lt = ligamentum teres,
   Vc = vena cava, Lc = caudate lobe,
   Lv = ligamentum venosum.

b The position of fingers 2 – 5 marks
   the course of the fissure for the ligamentum venosum.

c When the hand is supinated, the
   fingers trace around the superior
   pole of the caudate lobe (Lc).

KEY POINTS

**The vena cava separates the caudate
lobe from the right lobe of the liver.**

**The fissure of the ligamentum veno-
sum forms a true boundary surface
between the left lobe and caudate
lobe.**

the embryonic period. To help clarify the location of this fissure, a miniature
hand has been added to the drawing in Fig. 4.**78b**. The position of fingers 2
through 5 marks the course of the fissure between the left lobe and caudate
lobe. The hand has been supinated in Fig. 4.**78c**, moving the fingers around
the superior pole of the caudate lobe.

Review once again the location and course of the fissure. It runs on the inferior surface of the liver, passing upward and backward from the porta hepatis and separating the caudate lobe from the left lobe. The fissure thus forms
a true (curved) boundary surface between the left lobe and caudate lobe. Also,
analogous to the ligamentum teres in the lower part of the liver, it marks the
boundary surface between the anatomical left and right lobes in the upper
part of the liver.

Locating and scanning the fissure of the ligamentum venosum and the caudate lobe in transverse sections

Place the probe transversely on the upper abdomen, as close to the costal arch as possible. Identify the lumen of the vena cava and center it in the image. Angle the transducer slightly upward to scan into the liver. The fissure of the ligamentum venosum typically appears as a bright, echogenic arc, which is located above the caudate lobe and vena cava. Now angle the scan cephalad in small increments until the fissure disappears and the image is dominated by the large hepatic veins near the vena cava (Fig. 4.**79 a**). Then move the transducer caudad, scanning down the fissure to the porta hepatis (Fig. 4.**79 b, c**). Repeat this pass several times.

Fig. 4.**79**   *Scanning the fissure of the ligamentum venosum and the caudate lobe in transverse sections*

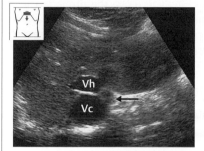
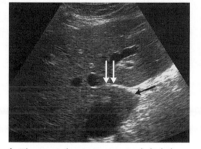
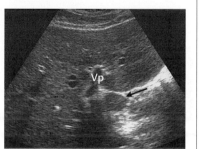

a Section through the superior pole of the caudate lobe (←).
Vc = vena cava, Vh = hepatic vein.

b The transducer was moved slightly caudad. This scan cuts the caudate lobe (←) at its maximum width. The ligamentum venosum (↓↓) is clearly defined.

c The transducer was moved lower. This scan cuts the inferior pole of the caudate lobe (←).
Vp = portal vein.

Scanning the fissure of the ligamentum venosum and caudate lobe in longitudinal sections

Obtain the familiar transverse section showing the fissure, caudate lobe, and vena cava. Rotate the transducer 90º while watching the screen. The fissure, which is broad in cross section, is now displayed longitudinally as a fine, echogenic line that has a typical, unmistakable appearance (Fig. 4.**80a,b**). Identify the four relevant structures: the fissure, caudate lobe, portal vein, and vena cava.

Now scan through the fissure in longitudinal sections. First, scan toward the left side until you see only the left lobe of the liver, then track slowly back to the right. First you will see a very small slice of the caudate lobe, which separates the fissure from the left lobe. Angle the scan farther to the right, and the section of the caudate lobe will become larger. Keep it centered in the image to define as much of the fissure as possible, which forms a bright band extending from the left to the right side of the screen. The vena cava comes into view posteriorly (Fig. 4.**80c**). As you move the probe farther to the right, the fissure disappears from the field of view, and the portal vein appears (Fig. 4.**80d**). Repeat this left-to-right pass several times. Acquire a feel for the extent of the caudate lobe. Figure 4.**81** shows an enlarged caudate lobe in a cirrhotic liver.

Fig. 4.80   *Defining the fissure of the ligamentum venosum and caudate lobe in longitudinal sections*

a Longitudinal section through the caudate lobe (Lc), ligamentum venosum (Lv), and ligamentum teres (Lt). Vp = portal vein, Lf = falciform ligament.

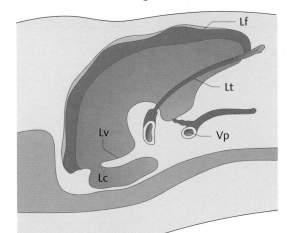

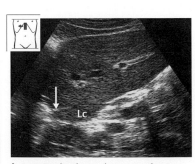

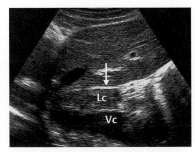

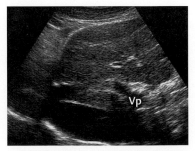

b Longitudinal scan between the aorta and vena cava demonstrates a small section of the caudate lobe (Lc) and fissure (↓).

c The transducer was moved a short distance to the right. The section of the caudate lobe (Lc) becomes larger. The fissure (↓) is clearly visualized. The vena cava (Vc) is seen posterior to the caudate lobe.

d The transducer was moved farther to the right. The fissure disappears from the image, and a section of the portal vein (Vp) comes into view.

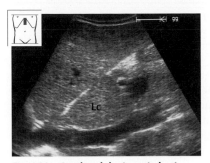

Fig. 4.81 **Caudate lobe in a cirrhotic liver.** Cirrhosis is often associated with conspicuous enlargement of the caudate lobe (Lc).

Hepatic veins and segmental anatomy of the liver

You have seen how the liver is divided into lobes. It is also subdivided into segments in a somewhat more complicated scheme. The main sonographic landmarks that define the boundaries of these segments are the hepatic veins, portal vein branches, fissures, vena cava, and gallbladder.

You know the three main hepatic veins: the left, middle, and right hepatic veins. They all converge at the posterosuperior border of the liver, where they empty into the vena cava (Fig. 4.**82 a**). They divide the liver into a lateral, medial, anterior, and posterior segment. Figure 4.**82 b** demonstrates the sonographic anatomy in transverse section.

Fig. 4.82 **Anatomy of the hepatic veins**

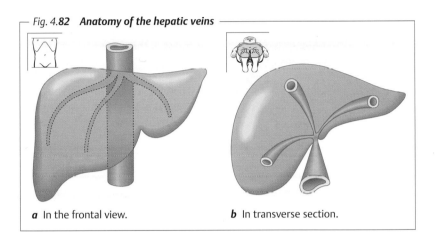

a In the frontal view.

b In transverse section.

The hepatic veins are the structures that mark the segmental boundaries in the upper portion of the liver (Fig. 4.**83**).

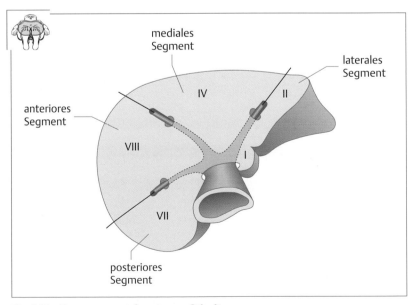

Fig. 4.83 **Upper segmental anatomy of the liver.**

➤ The left hepatic vein divides the lateral and medial segments.
➤ The middle hepatic vein divides the medial and anterior segments.
➤ The right hepatic vein divides the anterior and posterior segments.

The segments are divided into subsegments, which are numbered as follows:
Cranial subsegment of the lateral segment: II.
Cranial subsegment of the medial segment: IV.
Cranial subsegment of the anterior segment: VIII.
Cranial subsegment of the posterior segment: VII.
The familiar caudate lobe is considered a separate segment and is numbered I.

In the lower portion of the liver, additional segmentation landmarks are needed because the hepatic veins run backward and upward from the periphery of the organ to terminate at the vena cava, which is posterior and superior. As a result, the hepatic veins are small and arborized in the lower, peripheral portions of the liver.

The segmentation landmarks in the lower part of the liver are as follows:
➤ The ligamentum teres divides the lateral and medial segments.
➤ The gallbladder–vena cava line divides the medial and anterior segments.
➤ The right portal vein branch divides the anterior and posterior segments (Fig. 4.**84**).

The subsegment are numbered as follows:
Caudal subsegment of the lateral segment: III.
Caudal subsegment of the medial segment: IV.
Caudal subsegment of the anterior segment: V.
Caudal subsegment of the posterior segment: VI.

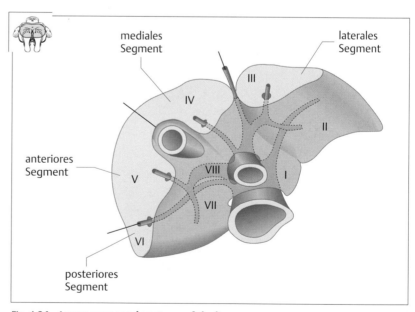

*Fig. 4.**84** **Lower segmental anatomy of the liver.***

This numbering system may seem confusing at first, but it does follow a certain order. The numbers are read counterclockwise along a double spiral that loops laterally downward, medially, anteriorly, posteriorly, and then back upward and anteriorly as shown in Fig. 4.**85**.

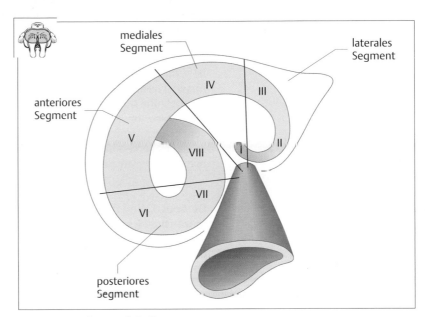

*Fig. 4.**85*** ***Numbering of the liver segments.***

Locating and defining the hepatic veins in transverse sections

The systematic survey of the hepatic veins begins with upper abdominal transverse scans. The scanning planes are shown schematically in Fig. 4.**86a**.

Position the probe transversely at the center of the upper abdomen. Angle upward and scan into the thoracic cage. Identify the circular cross section of the vena cava. By angling the probe gently up and down, you can locate the confluence of the hepatic veins immediately below the diaphragm (Fig. 4.**86b**). Remember this view, as it is the most reliable starting point for identifying the hepatic veins. Angle the transducer slightly downward. Observe how the sections of the hepatic veins move away from the vena cava in the image (Fig. 4.**86c**). Identify the individual hepatic veins.

Angle the transducer farther caudad and watch the sections of the hepatic veins move toward the periphery (Fig. 4.**86d**). Angle lower until the portal vein appears anterior to the vena cava and the right and left portal vein branches come into view. Repeat this sweep several times so that you can better appreciate the course of the hepatic veins.

Demonstrating the liver segments and subsegments in transverse sections

Next, image the hepatic veins at a level about midway between the superior border of the liver and the plane of the portal vein. Identify the hepatic segments and subsegments (Fig. 4.**86c**). Below, we will detail the techniques for surveying segments I through VIII in transverse sections.

Fig. 4.**86** *Defining the hepatic veins in transverse section*

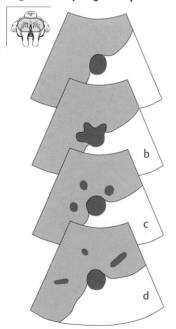

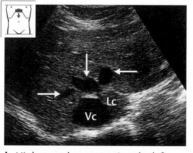

b High scan demonstrating the left (←), middle (↓) and right hepatic veins (→). Vc = vena cava, Lc = caudate lobe.

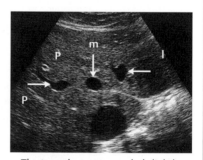

c The transducer was angled slightly caudad. The sections of the hepatic veins move away from the vena cava. l = lateral segment, m = medial segment, a = anterior segment, p = posterior segment.

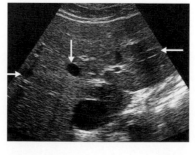

d The transducer was moved lower. The three hepatic veins move anteriorly and peripherally.

a Diagram of the scan planes at the level of the vena cava above image ***b*** and at the levels of images ***b–d***.

The lateral segment: subsegments II and III

Start with the lateral segment, which is separated from the medial segment by the left hepatic vein. Aim the scan slightly to the left so that this segment appears at the approximate center of the screen (Fig. 4.**87 a**). It is the number II segment in the upper part of the liver.

Now move the scan plane slowly caudad while observing the section of the left hepatic vein. As you do so, this section elongates and becomes a longitudinal section of the left hepatic vein extending into the left lobe (Fig. 4.**87 b**). Continue scanning lower (Fig. 4.**87 c**). You will see the left portal vein branch (Fig. 4.**87 d**), from which the now-familiar ligamentum teres originates. You have now reached the caudal subsegment of the lateral segment, designated as subsegment III. Scan down this subsegment to the inferior border of the liver (Fig. 4.**87 e, f**).

---

*Fig. 4.**87** **Scanning down the lateral segment in transverse sections***

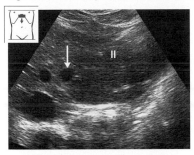

a High transverse scan through the lateral hepatic segment: subsegment II, left hepatic vein (↓).

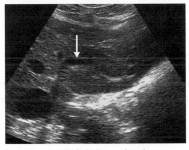

b Scan at a slightly lower level. The left hepatic vein (↓) extends into the left lobe.

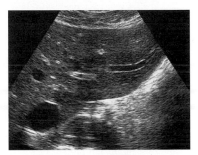

c Scan at a more distal level.

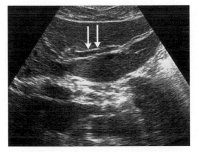

d Scan at the level of the left portal vein (↓↓).

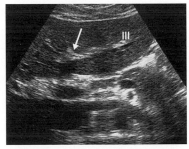

e The transducer was angled very slightly caudad. The ligamentum teres (←) comes into view. You are now scanning the caudal subsegment of the lateral segment, known as subsegment III.

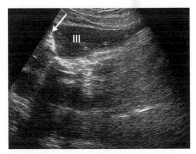

f Scan through subsegment III. Ligamentum teres (←).

The medial segment: subsegments I and IV

Scan transversely through the upper part of the liver. Identify the medial segment, which is located between the left and middle hepatic veins, and center it in the image. You will find the caudate lobe, designated as subsegment I, located anterior and slightly medial to the vena cava. Anterior to the caudate lobe is subsegment IV (Fig. 4.**88a**). Scan down this subsegment (Fig. 4.**88b**). You will see the trunk of the portal vein and its bifurcation into right and left branches appear near the bottom of the screen (Fig. 4.**88c**).

As you continue to scan lower, you will again recognize the ligamentum teres along with the interlobar fissure and the gallbladder, which appear to the right of the medial segment (Fig. 4.**88d, e**). Subsegment IV, then, is formed in this area by the quadrate lobe (Fig. 4.**88f**).

Fig. 4.88   *Scanning down the medial segment in transverse sections*

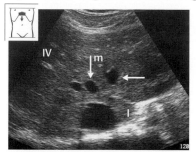

a Transverse scan through the medial segment of the liver (m), which is bounded by the left hepatic vein (←) and middle hepatic vein (↓). Subsegment IV is anterior, subsegment I (= the caudate lobe) is posterior.

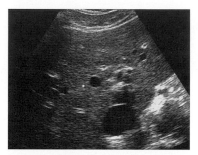

b The transducer was moved to a slightly lower level.

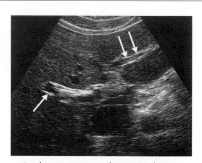

c As the scan moves lower, it shows part of the right portal vein branch (↑) and the left main branch (↓↓).

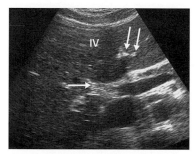

d Scanning farther downward reveals the quadrate lobe, which forms subsegment IV in this area. You also see the ligamentum teres (↓↓) and the interlobar fissure (→).

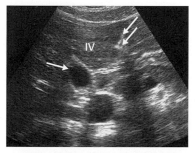

e As the scan continues to move caudad, the gallbladder (→) comes into view. Between it and the ligamentum teres (←←) is the quadrate lobe, which forms part of subsegment IV.

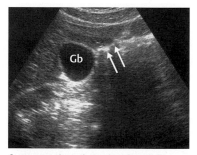

f Scan at the inferior border of the liver. The inferior border of the quadrate lobe (↑↑) is seen between the gallbladder (Gb) and ligamentum teres.

The anterior segment: subsegments VIII and V

Identify the anterior segment located between the middle and right hepatic veins. Center it in the image. To do this, you will have to place the transducer laterally on the right costal arch (Fig. 4.**89 a**). Trace the segment caudad (Fig. 4.**89 b, c**). Since you are holding the transducer on the descending margin of the right costal arch, it will be difficult for you to survey the entire segment. The cranial part of the anterior segment is subsegment VIII, and the caudal part is subsegment V.

*Fig. 4.**89*** **Scanning down the anterior segment in transverse sections**

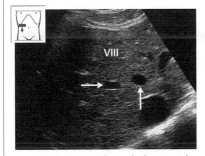

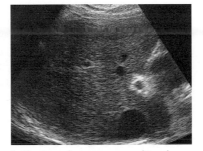

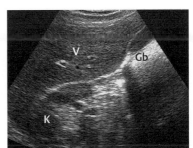

a Transverse scan through the cranial part of the anterior segment, subsegment VIII. This subsegment is bounded by the middle hepatic vein (↑) and right hepatic vein (→).

b The transducer was moved to a lower level. The scan plane lies approximately between subsegments VIII and V.

c Low scan of the anterior segment, passing through subsegment V. The kidney (K) appears on the left side of the screen, the gallbladder (Gb) on the right side.

The posterior segment: subsegments VII and VI

Scan the posterior segment from the lateral side by placing the transducer on the costal arch at about the level of the anterior axillary line. You must angle sharply upward toward the liver to demonstrate the confluence of the hepatic veins at the vena cava (Fig. 4.**90 a**). Scan down this segment in transverse sections (Fig. 4.**90 b, c**). The cranial part is subsegment VII, and the caudal part is subsegment VI.

*Fig. 4.**90*** **Scanning down the posterior segment in transverse sections**

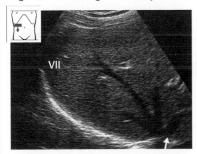

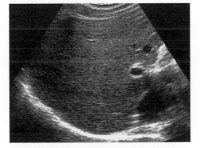

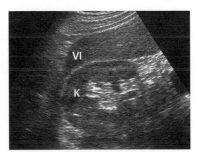

a High scan of the posterior segment through subsegment VII. Vena cava (↑).

b Scan at a level approximately between subsegments VII and VI.

c Low scan of the posterior segment through subsegment VI. K = kidney.

Locating and defining the hepatic veins in longitudinal sections and demonstrating the lower liver segments

You have seen that it is difficult to trace the hepatic veins into the periphery of the liver in transverse sections, simply because the vascular calibers become too small. You will now trace the hepatic veins in longitudinal sections.

Defining the left hepatic vein in longitudinal section

Start with the familiar transverse section displaying the inferior vena cava and hepatic veins (Fig. 4.**91 a**). Center over the left hepatic vein, and rotate the transducer until you see a longitudinal section of that vein near its termination (Fig. 4.**91 b**). Then trace the vein caudad in the longitudinal direction. While doing this, you will have to keep adjusting the transducer orientation to keep the vein in view. Trace the vein as far as you can toward the inferior border of the liver. Note the position of the lateral and medial segments. The left hepatic vein marks the boundary between the two segments, i.e., the medial segment lies in front of the image plane and the lateral segment lies behind the image plane. In Fig. 4.**91 c**, the left hepatic vein has been traced relatively far into the periphery of the liver. On the right side of the image, a branch of the left portal vein crosses over the vein and passes into the lower part of the lateral segment, designated as subsegment III.

Fig. 4.91 **Defining the left hepatic vein in longitudinal section**

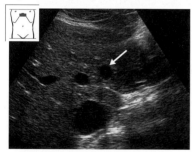 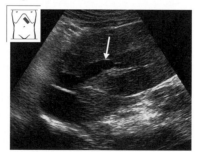 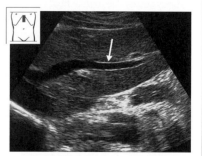

a Transverse scan through the left hepatic vein (↓), which is approximately centered in the image.

b The transducer was rotated almost to a longitudinal section over the left hepatic vein (↓).

c Longitudinal section of the left hepatic vein (↓). The lateral segment of the liver lies behind the image plane, the medial segment in front of it.

Defining the middle hepatic vein in longitudinal section

Image the middle hepatic vein transversely (Fig. 4.**92 a**), then turn the probe to a longitudinal scan. The vein enters the vena cava at an acute angle. Notice the structures that can be recognized in the image: the vena cava, into which the hepatic vein empties, and below it the right portal vein branch (Fig. 4.**92 b**). The medial hepatic segment is located behind the image plane, the anterior hepatic segment in front of it. The middle hepatic vein marks the boundary between the right and left lobes at this level. The caudal continuation of the middle hepatic vein leads out of the image plane and slightly toward the viewer. To trace its course, therefore, you have to move the transducer slightly lower and to the right. The gallbladder neck now lies against the right portal vein branch. At this point you have defined the vena cava–gallbladder plane, which marks the boundary between the left and right hepatic lobes in the lower portion of the liver. The anterior segment lies in front of the image plane, and the caudal part of the medial segment (the quadrate lobe) lies behind the image plane (Fig. 4.**92 c**).

Fig. 4.92   *Defining the middle hepatic vein in longitudinal section*

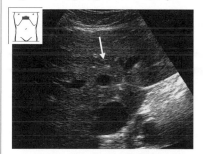

a Transverse scan through the middle hepatic vein (↓), which is approximately centered in the image.

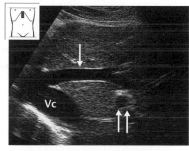

b The transducer was rotated to a longitudinal scan over the middle hepatic vein (↓). You see the entry of the vein into the vena cava (Vc). The right portal vein branch (↑↑) crosses inferior to the hepatic vein. The medial segment of the liver is located behind the image plane, the anterior segment in front of it.

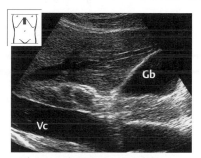

c The transducer was moved down along the middle hepatic vein. You see a section of the gallbladder (Gb) and a conspicuous section of the vena cava (Vc). The gallbladder–vena cava plane marks the boundary between the medial segment, which is behind the image plane, and the anterior segment, which is in front of the image plane.

Defining the right hepatic vein in longitudinal section

Like its left and middle counterparts, the right hepatic vein is imaged in longitudinal section and traced into the periphery of the liver. As we saw in the transverse sections, longitudinal scanning is made difficult by the intervening costal arch. The posterior hepatic segment lies in front of the image plane, the anterior segment behind it (Fig. 4.**93**).

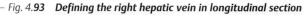

Fig. 4.93   **Defining the right hepatic vein in longitudinal section**

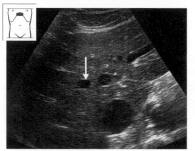
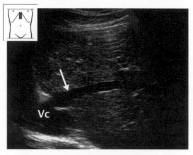
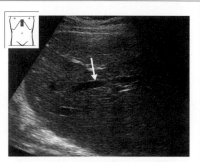

a Transverse scan through the right hepatic vein (↓).

b The transducer was rotated to a longitudinal scan. You see the entry of the right hepatic vein (↓) into the vena cava (Vc). The anterior segment of the liver is behind the image plane, the posterior segment in front of it.

c The transducer was moved caudad along the right hepatic vein (↓).

Surveying the liver segments in longitudinal sections

Now that you have systematically defined the hepatic veins, perform a complete longitudinal survey of the liver while giving attention to the segments and their boundaries (Fig. 4.**94**).

---

*Fig. 4.**94*** **Scanning across the liver in longitudinal sections, defining the segments and their boundaries**

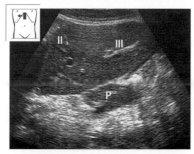

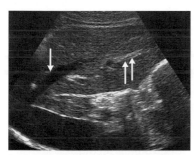

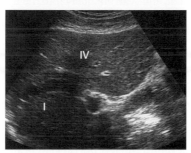

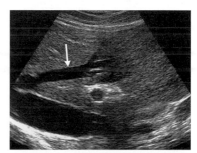

a Longitudinal scan through the lateral segment of the left lobe, subsegments II and III. P = pancreas.

b The transducer was moved slightly to the right. The left hepatic vein (↓) and ligamentum teres (↑↑) mark the boundary between the lateral and medial segments.

c Scan of the medial segment through subsegment IV, whose lower portion is the quadrate lobe, and subsegment I, which is the caudate lobe.

d Boundary between the medial and anterior segments, formed by the middle hepatic vein (↓).

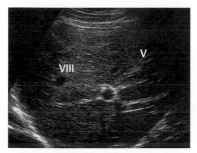

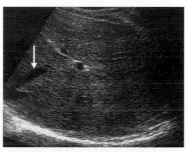

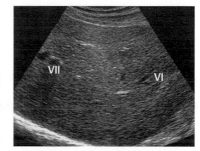

e Scan through the anterior segment, subsegments VIII and V.

f Boundary between the anterior and posterior segments, formed by the right hepatic vein (↓).

g Scan through the posterior segment, subsegments VII and VI.

The portal vein and its branches

In the previous section you learned the lobar and segmental anatomy of the liver and how to identify the hepatic lobes and segments using ligaments and veins as landmarks. In some places we assumed that you were familiar with the portal venous system. In this section you will review the portal vein and its branches and learn a systematic approach to scanning these structures.

The main trunk of the portal vein ascends at a slight angle from left to right, passing toward the costal arch. Upon entering the liver, it quickly divides into right and left main branches, which divide further into segmental branches. The portal vein and its branches are distributed to the center of the liver segments, accompanied by the hepatic arteries and bile ducts.

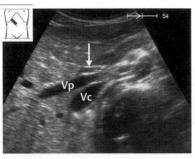

Fig. 4.95 Longitudinal section of the portal vein Vp = portal vein, Vc = vena cava, hepatic artery (↓).

Locating the portal vein

The anatomy of the porta hepatis is described in detail on p. 96 ff.

Place the transducer below the right costal arch, aligning it with the course of the portal vein. Ask the subject to take a deep breath, expanding the abdomen, and scan obliquely into the upper abdomen. Angle the transducer to locate the main trunk of the portal vein. Figure 4.95 shows the typical appearance of the vessel.

Image the portal vein in a plane that defines the longest possible segment. When you have done this, you will also have an oblique section of the vena cava and hepatic artery. The three-dimensional course of the portal vein and its branches is very difficult to appreciate in oblique sections. For this reason, it is best to define these structures in longitudinal and transverse sections.

TIP

To define the course of the portal vein, have the subject inflate the abdomen, and then scan obliquely into the upper abdomen.

Defining the left portal vein branch in longitudinal sections

Locate the portal vein in an upper abdominal oblique scan as described above. While watching the screen, rotate the transducer over the portal vein to a longitudinal scan. As you do this, observe how the elongated section of the portal vein becomes round or oval. The typical appearance is shown in Fig. 4.96.

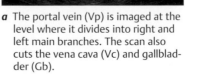

Fig. 4.96 Longitudinal scan of the portal vein

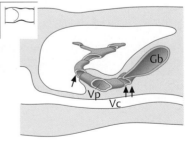

a The portal vein (Vp) is imaged at the level where it divides into right and left main branches. The scan also cuts the vena cava (Vc) and gallbladder (Gb).

b Diagram shows additional sections that are obtained by moving the transducer to the left. Notice that the sections of the intrahepatic left portal vein (↑) and extrahepatic portal vein (↑↑) lie in the same image plane.

From this starting point (Fig. 4.**97 a**), slide the transducer to the left in small, parallel increments. Observe how the section of the portal vein changes, becoming more elongated and then dividing as the scan moves farther left. Picture what this means: The vascular section that appears on the right (caudal) represents the confluence of the superior mesenteric and splenic veins, from which the portal vein arises and inclines toward the porta hepatis from the midline. The section seen at upper left (cranial) corresponds to the left portal vein branch, which initially passes upward, anteriorly, and to the left (Fig. 4.**97 b**). From now on, focus your attention entirely on this vascular section. Keep moving the transducer to the left in small steps and observe the course of the left portal vein branch: It continues in a typical arch that runs forward and then downward (Fig. 4.**97 c**). This portion of the left branch is called the umbilical part. At this level you see the now-familiar ligamentum teres, which, as you recall, runs from the left portal vein branch to the umbilicus. If you now move the transducer a little more to the left, you will see the left portal vein splitting into segmental branches (Fig. 4.**97 d**). Follow the sections of these branches into the periphery (Fig. 4.**97 e, f**).

---

*Fig. 4.***97** *Defining the left portal vein branch in longitudinal sections*

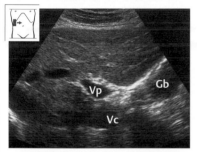

a Longitudinal scan through the portal vein (Vp). Notice the oblong shape of the section. Gb = gallbladder, Vc = vena cava.

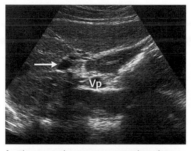

b The transducer was moved to the left. At this point the left main branch of the portal vein (→) is slightly anterior and cranial to the portal trunk (Vp), which is still in the image.

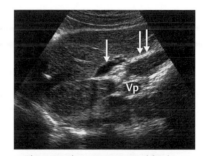

c The transducer was moved farther to the left. The left portal vein branch now curves downward (↓). You can see the ligamentum teres (↓↓) and portal vein (Vp).

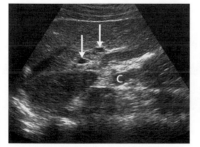

d The transducer was moved farther to the left. The left portal vein branch has divided into segmental branches (↓). C = confluence.

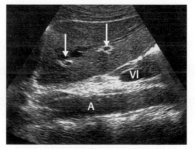

e As the transducer is moved farther to the left, the two portal vein branches move apart (↓). Vl = splenic vein, A = aorta.

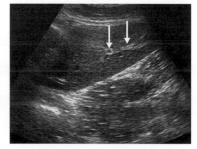

f Longitudinal scan through the peripheral part of the left lobe. Fine portal venous branches (↓) can still be seen.

Defining the left portal vein branch in transverse sections

Understanding the appearance of the left portal vein branch in transverse sections requires a greater ability to visualize in three dimensions compared with longitudinal sections. Recall that the left portal vein branch first turns superiorly and anteriorly and then curves back downward (Fig. 4.**98 a**).

Place the probe transversely over the portal vein and identify the portal trunk (Fig. 4.**98 b**). Then move the probe cephalad. Observe the bifurcation of the trunk into the left and right branches (Fig. 4.**98 c**). Keep your eye on the left portal vein branch and see how it projects into the left lobe. Now move the scan higher to define the apex of the left branch (Fig. 4.**98 d**). If you scan still higher from this point, the left branch will disappear from the image.

Fig. 4.98   Defining the left portal vein branch in transverse sections

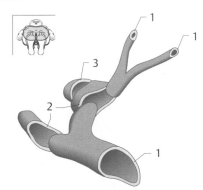

a The left portal vein branch first runs upward and anteriorly and then turns down toward the viewer. Three typical planes of section are encountered as the scan moves cephalad:
Plane 1: the extrahepatic portal vein with anterior intrahepatic branches.
Plane 2: the division into the left and right branches.
Plane 3: the apex of the left portal vein branch.

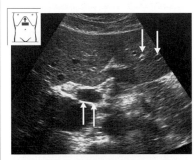

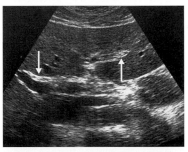

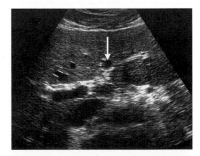

b Scan corresponding to plane 1 in **a**. Section of the portal trunk (↑↑). Sections of portal vein branches (↓) are visible in the periphery of the liver.

c Scan corresponding to plane 2 in **a**. The transducer was moved slightly cephalad. The portal vein divides into the right (↓) and left (↑) main branches.

d Scan corresponding to plane 3 in **a**. The transducer was moved farther cephalad, demonstrating the apex of the left portal vein branch (↓).

Defining the right portal vein branch in longitudinal sections

The technique for scanning the right portal vein branch is analogous to that for the left branch. Locate the portal vein in the upper abdominal oblique scan and rotate to a longitudinal scan while watching the screen (Fig. 4.**99 a**, **b**). Move the transducer to the right in small increments. Observe the section of the right portal vein branch as the vena cava disappears from the image. The section of the vein will move slightly downward (posteriorly) in the image. As you continue to move the transducer, you will see the right portal vein divide into two branches (Fig. 4.**99 c**). One branch continues superiorly while the other branch runs inferiorly. Trace the sections into the periphery of the right hepatic lobe (Fig. 4.**99 d**).

Fig. 4.**99**   *Defining the right portal vein branch in longitudinal sections*

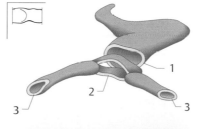

a *Plane 1:* the right portal vein branch at the level of the gallbladder–vena cava plane.
Plane 2: division of the right main branch into peripheral branches.
Plane 3: continuation of the peripheral branches.

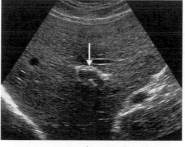

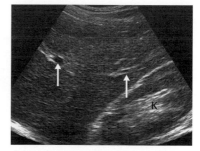

b Scan corresponding to plane 1 in ***a***. Section of the right portal vein branch (↓) at the level of the gallbladder–vena cava plane. Vc = vena cava, Gb = gallbladder.

c Scan corresponding to plane 2 in ***a***. The transducer was moved slightly to the right. The right portal vein branch is beginning to divide (↓).

d Scan corresponding to plane 3 in ***a***. The transducer was moved farther to the right. This is a longitudinal section through the periphery of the liver, cutting the peripheral branches of the right portal vein (↑). K = kidney.

Defining the right portal vein branch in transverse sections

The course of the right portal vein branch, like that of the left branch, can be difficult to define and interpret, especially in transverse sections. Remember: the right portal vein branch first runs laterally and then bifurcates into a superior and inferior branch.

Position the probe transversely over the portal vein (Fig. 4.**100a, b**) and slide it cephalad in small increments. Observe how the right portal vein branch passes into the right lobe of the liver (Fig. 4.**100c**). Angle the transducer farther upward, and you will see the oblong section of the right branch change to a round cross section (Fig. 4.**100d**).

Fig. 4.100   Defining the right portal vein branch in transverse sections

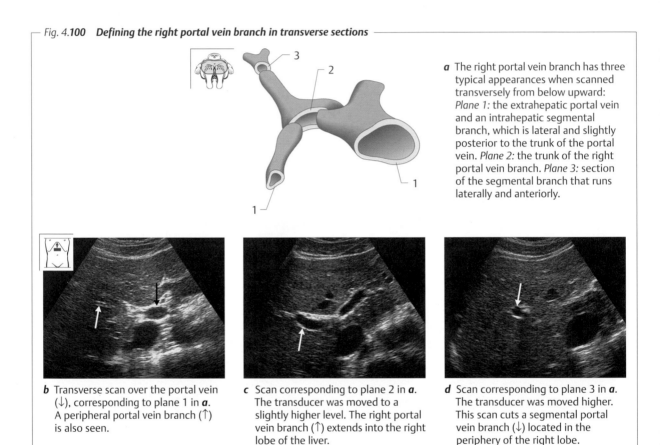

a The right portal vein branch has three typical appearances when scanned transversely from below upward: *Plane 1:* the extrahepatic portal vein and an intrahepatic segmental branch, which is lateral and slightly posterior to the trunk of the portal vein. *Plane 2:* the trunk of the right portal vein branch. *Plane 3:* section of the segmental branch that runs laterally and anteriorly.

b Transverse scan over the portal vein (↓), corresponding to plane 1 in **a**. A peripheral portal vein branch (↑) is also seen.

c Scan corresponding to plane 2 in **a**. The transducer was moved to a slightly higher level. The right portal vein branch (↑) extends into the right lobe of the liver.

d Scan corresponding to plane 3 in **a**. The transducer was moved higher. This scan cuts a segmental portal vein branch (↓) located in the periphery of the right lobe.

Anatomical Relationships

━━━━━━━━━━━ LEARNING GOALS
➤ Define the relationship of the liver to neighboring organs and structures, particularly the heart, stomach, pancreas, aorta, vena cava, gallbladder, right kidney, and porta hepatis.

The liver is the dominant organ of the upper abdomen, occupying the anterior part of the right upper abdomen and extending a considerable distance into the left upper abdomen. To understand the relationships of the liver, it is helpful to divide the organ into three zones: a left portion, central portion, and right portion (Fig. 4.**101**).

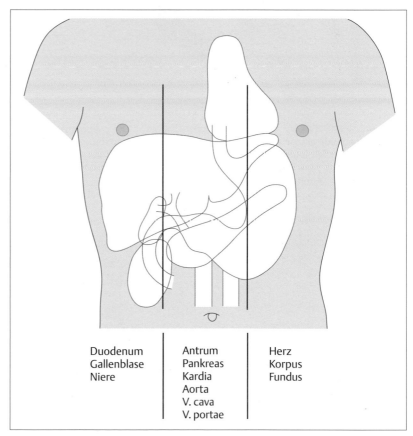

Duodenum	Antrum	Herz
Gallenblase	Pankreas	Korpus
Niere	Kardia	Fundus
	Aorta	
	V. cava	
	V. portae	

*Fig. 4.**101*** ***Relationships of the liver to other organs.***

Relationship of the left portion of the liver to the heart and stomach

The left border of the hepatic left lobe lies between the chest wall (anterior), the heart (superior and anterior), and the stomach (posterior and lateral) (Fig. 4.**102**).

Fig. 4.**102**   *Relationships of the left portion of the liver*

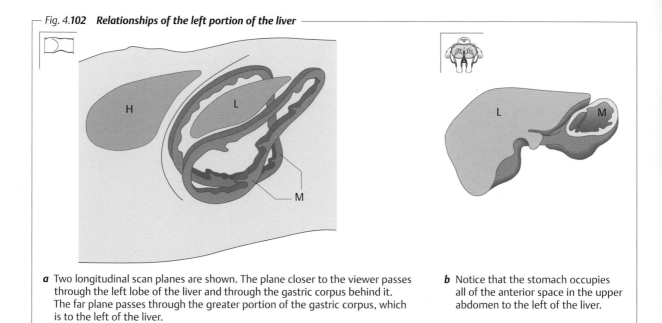

a Two longitudinal scan planes are shown. The plane closer to the viewer passes through the left lobe of the liver and through the gastric corpus behind it. The far plane passes through the greater portion of the gastric corpus, which is to the left of the liver.

b Notice that the stomach occupies all of the anterior space in the upper abdomen to the left of the liver.

Defining the relationship of the left portion of the liver to the heart and stomach

Place the probe transversely on the upper abdomen to the left of the midline, as for scanning the left lobe. Identify the homogeneous texture of the liver in the left half of the image, contrasting it with the nonhomogeneous pattern of the stomach on the right side of the image. Then angle the probe sharply upward and watch the pulsating heart come into view. You will observe a typical arrangement with the liver above, the heart below, and the stomach to the right (Fig. 4.**103a**). Please note the direction of the scan for this section. The liver is narrow in its craniocaudal dimension, but because it is scanned obliquely, a relatively large transverse section is seen (Fig. 4.**104a**). The spatial relationships in this view are somewhat difficult to understand and are explained below.

When the probe is placed transversely on the body surface at a perpendicular angle, the examiner is viewing the body section from below upward. But when the transducer is tilted to a very low tangential angle, the orientation changes; the examiner is now looking from back to front. The top of the image is inferior, and the bottom of the image is superior. Put more simply, the examiner is viewing the scan from back to front with the body turned upside down (Fig. 4.**104b**).

KEY POINT

With a tangential scan, the sonographer is viewing the section from back to front as if the body were turned "upside down."

Fig. 4.103 Relationships of liver, heart, stomach – transverse and longitudinal scans

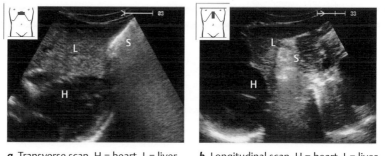

a Transverse scan. H = heart, L = liver, S = stomach.

b Longitudinal scan. H = heart, L = liver, S = stomach.

Fig. 4.104 Tangential scanning of the liver and heart

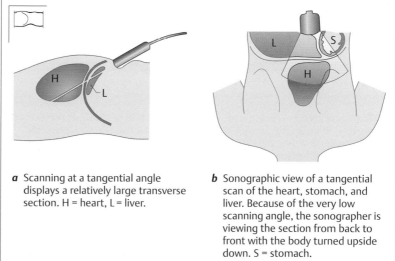

a Scanning at a tangential angle displays a relatively large transverse section. H = heart, L = liver.

b Sonographic view of a tangential scan of the heart, stomach, and liver. Because of the very low scanning angle, the sonographer is viewing the section from back to front with the body turned upside down. S = stomach.

Relationship of the central portion of the liver to the vena cava, stomach, and pancreas

The vena cava is in contact with the posterior surface of the liver, specifically with the caudate lobe (Fig. 4.**105**). Below this area of contact are the pancreas and stomach.

Fig. 4.**105**   *Relationships of the central portion of the liver*

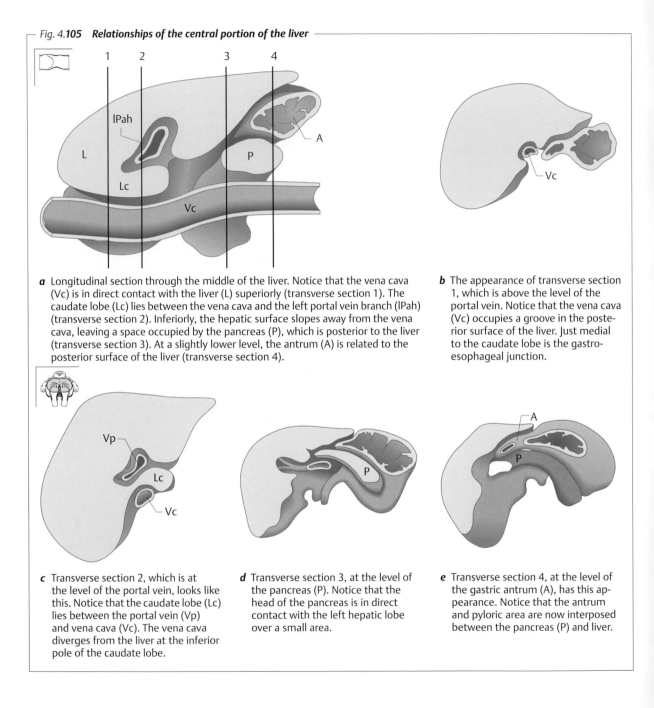

a Longitudinal section through the middle of the liver. Notice that the vena cava (Vc) is in direct contact with the liver (L) superiorly (transverse section 1). The caudate lobe (Lc) lies between the vena cava and the left portal vein branch (lPah) (transverse section 2). Inferiorly, the hepatic surface slopes away from the vena cava, leaving a space occupied by the pancreas (P), which is posterior to the liver (transverse section 3). At a slightly lower level, the antrum (A) is related to the posterior surface of the liver (transverse section 4).

b The appearance of transverse section 1, which is above the level of the portal vein. Notice that the vena cava (Vc) occupies a groove in the posterior surface of the liver. Just medial to the caudate lobe is the gastroesophageal junction.

c Transverse section 2, which is at the level of the portal vein, looks like this. Notice that the caudate lobe (Lc) lies between the portal vein (Vp) and vena cava (Vc). The vena cava diverges from the liver at the inferior pole of the caudate lobe.

d Transverse section 3, at the level of the pancreas (P). Notice that the head of the pancreas is in direct contact with the left hepatic lobe over a small area.

e Transverse section 4, at the level of the gastric antrum (A), has this appearance. Notice that the antrum and pyloric area are now interposed between the pancreas (P) and liver.

Defining the relationship of the central portion of the liver to the vena cava and cardia in transverse sections

Demonstrate the liver, vena cava, and aorta in a high upper abdominal transverse scan, displaying all three structures in one image (Fig. 4.**106a**). Move the transducer caudad, and repeat this craniocaudal pass several times (Fig. 4.**106b**, **c**). Identify the vena cava, aorta, and caudate lobe (which you already know), and then identify the gastric cardia, which is directly anterior to the aorta.

Fig. 4.106 **Relationships of the liver, vena cava, and cardia in transverse scans**

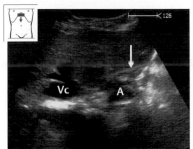
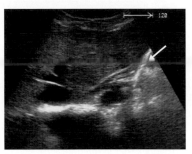
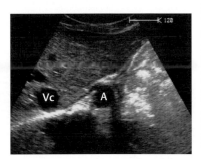

a High transverse scan demonstrates the aorta (A) and vena cava (Vc) with the gastroesophageal junction (↓) above.

b The transducer was moved slightly lower. The cardia is opening into the body of the stomach (↓).

c Transverse scan at a more caudal level.

Defining the relationship of the central portion of the liver to the vena cava and cardia in longitudinal sections

Now, while watching the monitor, rotate the transducer over the aorta to a longitudinal scan (Fig. 4.**107a**). Identify the following structures: liver, cardia, and aorta. Angle the transducer slightly to the right and define the caudate lobe and vena cava (Figs. 4.**107b**, **c**).

Fig. 4.107 **Relationship of the liver, vena cava, and cardia in longitudinal scans**

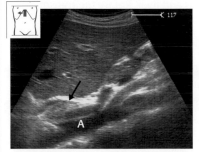
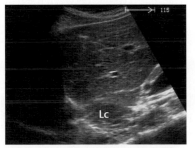
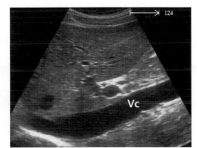

a Longitudinal scan over the aorta (A). The gastroesophageal junction (↓) can be recognized between the aorta and liver.

b The transducer was moved a little to the right. The caudate lobe (Lc) is clearly visualized.

c The transducer was moved farther to the right, defining the vena cava in longitudinal section. The vena cava is in contact with the liver at this level. Vc = vena cava.

Defining the relationship of the central portion of the liver to the pancreas in transverse and longitudinal sections

Position the transducer for an upper abdominal transverse scan. Identify the pancreas, using the splenic vein as a landmark (Fig. 4.**108 a**). Angle the probe back and forth several times in a craniocaudal sweep. Then rotate the probe under vision to a longitudinal scan and identify the liver, pancreas, and splenic vein (Fig. 4.**108 b**).

Fig. 4.108   Relationship of the liver and pancreas – transverse and longitudinal scans

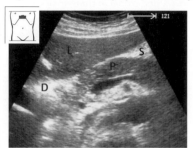 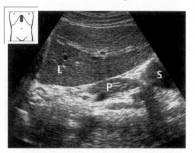

a Notice that in the transverse scan, a short segment of the body of the pancreas (P) directly borders the liver (L). The stomach (S) lies between the pancreas and liver on the right side of the image, and the duodenum (D) lies between the pancreas and liver on the left side of the image.

b Longitudinal scan. L = liver, S = stomach, P = pancreas

Defining the relationship of the central portion of the liver to the gastric antrum in transverse and longitudinal sections

Place the probe transversely at the center of the upper abdomen (Fig. 4.**109 a**) and identify the pancreas using the technique described above. Observe the section of the gastric antrum on the right side of the image. Now angle the transducer caudad and observe the following: the section of the antrum intervenes like a wedge between the pancreas and liver. Rotate the transducer to a longitudinal plane (Fig. 4.**109 b**). Scan through the imaged region in a fan-shaped pattern and identify the following structures: the liver, antrum, and pancreas.

Fig. 4.109   Relationship of the liver and antrum – transverse and longitudinal scans

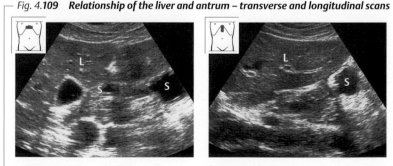

a Transverse scan. L = liver, S = antrum of stomach.

b Longitudinal scan. L = liver, S = stomach.

Relationship of the right portion of the liver to the gallbladder, duodenum, and kidney

The right portion of the liver is related directly to the visceral surface of the kidney, the gallbladder, and the duodenum (Fig. 4.**110 a**). Figure 4.**110 b, c** show the appearance of these relationships in upper abdominal transverse scans.

---

*Fig. 4.**110** Relationships of the right portion of the liver*

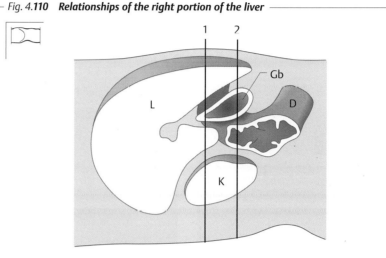

a In this longitudinal section, notice that the kidney (K) extends to a relatively high level posterior to the liver. Part of the right lobe of the liver (L) and part of the duodenum (D) are interposed between the kidney and gallbladder (Gb).

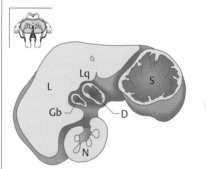 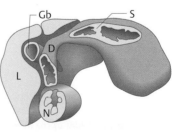

b High transverse section through the neck of the gallbladder neck and the upper pole of the kidney (level 1 in **a**). Notice that the section through the roof of the duodenal bulb (D) is medial to the gallbladder (Gb). The duodenal bulb adjoins the quadrate lobe (Lq) posteriorly. Part of the right lobe of the liver is interposed between the gallbladder and kidney (N). The kidney impresses the posterior surface of the right lobe. S = stomach.

c Low transverse section through the gallbladder fundus and lower pole of the kidney (N) (level 2 in **a**). Note that the duodenum (D) is posterior to the gallbladder (Gb). The duodenum borders the medial aspect of the right lobe of the liver (L) and the anterior surface of the right kidney. S = stomach.

Defining the relationships of the right portion of the liver to the gallbladder, duodenum, and right kidney in transverse sections

Place the transducer to the right of the midline for a high transverse scan. Position the cross section of the gallbladder at the approximate center of the image. Identify the following structures: liver, gallbladder, and vena cava (Fig. 4.**111 a**). Scan caudad in small steps and then back up to the initial level while you note the following relationships. The gallbladder occupies a depression in the inferior surface of the liver. At the level of the gallbladder neck, the upper part of the duodenum directly borders the liver medially. Lower down, at the level of the gallbladder fundus, the duodenum is interposed laterally and posteriorly between the gallbladder and vena cava (Fig. 4.**111 b**). It now abuts the liver lateral to the gallbladder. If imaging conditions are good, you can also recognize the cross section of the kidney farther laterally and posteriorly (Fig. 4.**111 c**).

Fig. 4.111   Relationships of the liver, gallbladder, duodenum, and right kidney in transverse scans

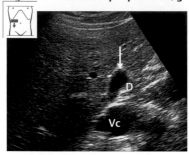

a Transverse scan through the gallbladder (↓), duodenum (D), and vena cava (Vc).

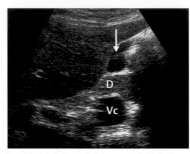

b The transducer was moved slightly caudad. The duodenum (D) comes between the gallbladder (↓) and vena cava (Vc).

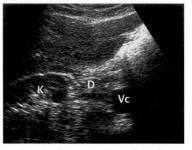

c The transducer was moved to a lower level. You see the vena cava (Vc), kidney (K), and duodenum (D).

Defining the relationship of the right portion of the liver to the gallbladder, duodenum, and right kidney in longitudinal sections

Demonstrate the liver in a longitudinal scan over the vena cava. Identify the following structures: liver, vena cava, and the duodenum wedged between them (Fig. 4.**112 a**). Move the transducer slightly to the right, and identify the gallbladder (Fig. 4.**112 b**). Slide the transducer farther to the right, and you can identify the kidney if scanning conditions are good (Fig. 4.**112 c**).

Fig. 4.112   Relationships of the liver, gallbladder, duodenum, and right kidney in longitudinal scans

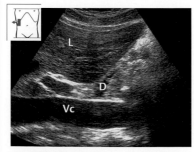

a Longitudinal scan over the vena cava (Vc). The duodenum (D) is seen between the vena cava and liver (L).

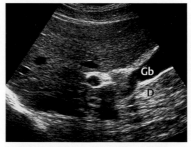

b The transducer was moved a little to the right. Now the gallbladder (Gb) lies between the duodenum (D) and liver.

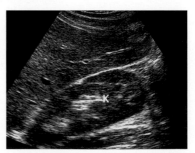

c The transducer was moved farther to the right. The kidney (K) lies against the inferior border of the liver.

Ascites

Even a small amount of ascites can be detected with ultrasound as a thin fluid layer outlining the liver. An initial fluid collection may be visible only in Morrison's pouch (hepatorenal recess), which is the lowest point in the right upper abdomen in the supine patient (Fig. 4.**113 a, b**). As the fluid collection increases, it also fills the subphrenic space (Fig. 4.**113 c**).

Fig. 4.*113*   *Ascites in Morrison's pouch and the subphrenic space*

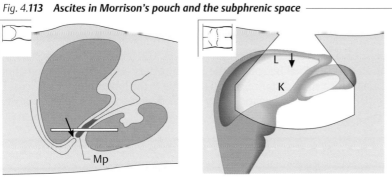

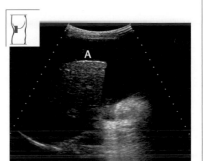

a Morrison's pouch (Rh) is the lowest point in the right upper abdomen. The triangular ligament (↓) separates Morrison's pouch from the subphrenic space. The two spaces communicate with each other lateral to the triangular ligament, or out-of-plane towards the viewer. The white line indicates the scan plane that is used to detect small amounts of ascites.

b Representation of the scan plane. When scanning in this plane, the examiner is viewing the body section from behind. Because the subject is supine, the fluid collects at the lowest point (↓). L = liver, K = kidney.

c Pronounced ascites (A). Fluid also fills the subphrenic space.

5 Porta hepatis

━━━━━━━━━━━━━━━━━━━ **LEARNING GOAL**

➤ Identify and evaluate the vascular structures about the porta hepatis.

The porta hepatis can be a challenging region for the ultrasound novice. But by working systematically to learn this region, you should be able to identify and evaluate its vascular structures without difficulty.

Three vascular structures enter or leave the liver at the porta hepatis: the portal vein, the hepatic artery, and the common hepatic duct. The inferior vena cava runs distal to this triad (Fig. 5.**1**). The bile duct lies approximately on the longitudinal body axis. The hepatic artery and portal vein run almost parallel for a short distance, at a slight angle to the longitudinal body axis. The initial portion of the hepatic artery is almost perpendicular to this body axis (Fig. 5.**2**).

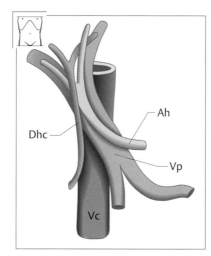

Fig. 5.1 **The vessels of the porta hepatis: bile duct (Dhc), hepatic artery (Ah), portal vein (Vp), and vena cava (Vc).** This diagram is familiar to you from anatomy. Take note of the following relationships: the bile duct and hepatic artery are anterior to the portal vein; the bile duct is lateral to the hepatic artery and portal vein.

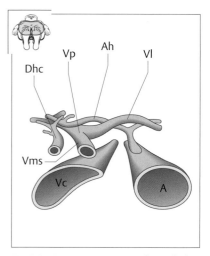

Fig. 5.**2** **Transverse section through the porta hepatis.** Dhc = common hepatic duct, Vp = portal vein, Vms = superior mesenteric vein, Vl = splenic vein, Ah = hepatic artery, Vc = vena cava, A = aorta.

Organ Boundaries: Identifying the Vessels in the Porta Hepatis

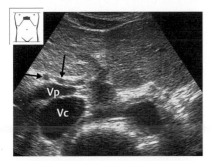

Fig. 5.3 Transverse scan at the level of the porta hepatis. You should positively identify two vessels at this level: the vena cava (Vc) posteriorly and the adjacent portal vein (Vp) anteriorly. The vascular sections in front of the portal vein are initially difficult to identify: the hepatic artery (↓) and common hepatic duct (→).

The key sonographic landmark for the portal vessels is the portal vein itself. An upper abdominal transverse scan can define this vessel in its course anterior to the vena cava. It is helpful to have the subject take a deep breath, expanding the abdomen. Figure 5.**3** shows the typical ultrasound appearance.

Vena cava and portal vein

These vessels can be identified by applying a simple technical principle. First confirm the identity of the vena cava.

Identifying the vena cava

Define the vena cava and portal vein in cross section as shown in Fig. 5.3. While watching the screen, rotate the transducer to a longitudinal scan over the vena cava so that you can positively identify that vessel. Then return to the initial position over the portal vein and vena cava.

Identifying the portal vein

Confirm your identification of the portal vein by rotating the transducer clockwise from the transverse plane (Fig. 5.**4a**) until you see a longitudinal section of the portal vein (Fig. 5.**4b**). Move the transducer a short distance medially, and you will have no trouble recognizing the terminal portion of the splenic vein (Fig. 5.**4c**). Trace that vessel back to the portal vein.

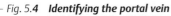
Fig. 5.4 Identifying the portal vein

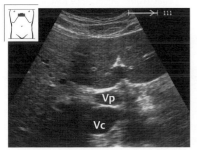

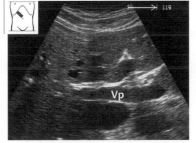

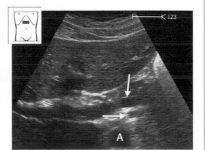

a Transverse scan through the vena cava (Vc) and portal vein (Vp).

b The transducer was rotated clockwise to obtain a longitudinal section of the portal vein (Vp).

c The transducer was moved a short distance medially along the portal vein, which is continuous with the splenic vein (↓). Superior mesenteric artery (→), A = aorta.

Hepatic artery and bile duct

The main problem in examining the porta hepatis is in distinguishing between the hepatic artery and the bile duct. This should not be difficult, however, if you are familiar with the anatomy of the region.

Since the cystic duct cannot be positively identified with ultrasound, we will refer to the common hepatic duct and common bile duct collectively as the bile duct.

Recall that the hepatic artery curves across the vena cava to the celiac trunk, while the bile duct runs almost longitudinally, parallel to the vena cava, toward the head of the pancreas. This means that you can obtain a longitudinal section of the hepatic artery by rotating the transducer counterclockwise.

Identifying the hepatic artery

Place the transducer obliquely along the right costal arch, and image the portal vein in longitudinal section as described above under "Identifying the portal vein" (Fig. 5.**5a**). Now rotate the transducer counterclockwise to an upper abdominal transverse scan. You will see the hepatic artery just above the portal vein, coursing left toward the aorta (Fig. 5.**5b**). Trace the longitudinal section of the hepatic artery to the celiac trunk and then back to the porta hepatis (Fig. 5.**5c**).

Fig. 5.5 **Identifying the hepatic artery**

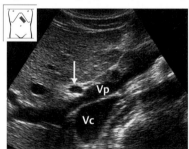

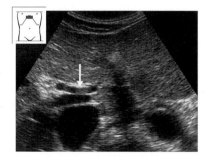

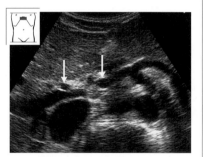

a Longitudinal section of the portal vein (Vp) with a cross section of the hepatic artery (↓). Vc = vena cava.

b The transducer was rotated counterclockwise to an upper abdominal transverse scan. This gives an elongated section of the hepatic artery (↓).

c The transducer was rotated further. The hepatic artery merges with the celiac trunk. Because of its curvature, the hepatic artery is cut twice by the scan (↓).

Identifying the bile duct

Image the portal vein again (Fig. 5.**6a**). Rotate the transducer to an approximate longitudinal scan. If scanning conditions are good, you can now identify the bile duct anterior and inferior to the imaged section of the portal vein. The bile duct runs parallel to the vena cava toward the head of the pancreas (Fig. 5.**6b, c**).

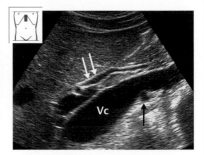

— Fig. 5.**6** *Identifying the bile duct* —

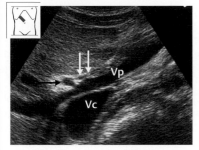

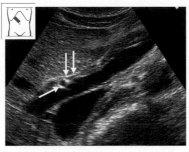

a Longitudinal section of the portal vein (Vp). The hepatic artery (→) is well-defined. The bile duct (↓↓) is faintly visible. Vc = vena cava.

b With slight clockwise rotation of the transducer, the section of the bile duct is more clearly defined and the section of the hepatic artery (→) is more rounded. Note that the hepatic artery impresses the bile duct (↓↓), not the other way around!

c The transducer was rotated to a longitudinal scan. You can clearly recognize the longitudinal section of the bile duct (↓↓), which passes into the head of the pancreas. You also see the right renal artery (↑), which crosses behind the vena cava (Vc).

Transverse and longitudinal survey of the porta hepatis

The method described above has proven very effective for routine examinations of the porta hepatis. Below we shall revisit the porta hepatis and explore it systematically in transverse and longitudinal scans in order to understand the exact spatial relationships of the vessels to one another.

Defining the porta hepatis in transverse sections

Figure 5.**2** showed you the basic appearance of the portal vessels in transverse section. The diagram in Fig. 5.**7** shows their relationships in somewhat greater detail.

*Fig. 5.***7** *Transverse section just below the porta hepatis.* The plane of section passes through the duodenum (D), papilla (P), gastric antrum (S), superior mesenteric vein (Vms), vena cava (Vc), and aorta (A). Only one slice each was shown for the duodenum and stomach in order to demonstrate the vessels at higher levels. Al = splenic artery. Notice that the portal vein (Vp), hepatic artery (Ah), and bile duct (Dhc) are initially close together. Above the splenic vein (Vl), the hepatic artery curves to the left toward the aorta. As the bile duct descends from the porta hepatis, it turns toward the longitudinal body axis.

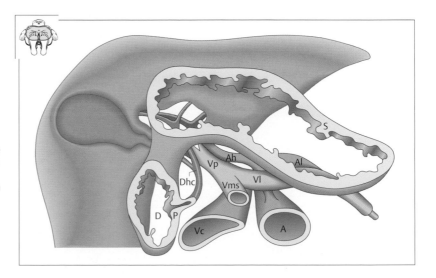

Place the transducer in the familiar upper abdominal transverse scan position, and identify the vena cava and portal vein. When you see both vessels close together, you can be almost certain that the scan also cuts the hepatic artery and bile duct, even if you cannot positively identify them. You also know that the hepatic artery turns to the left while the bile duct descends parallel to the vena cava (Fig. 5.**8a**). In thin patients, you will usually be able to identify the hepatic artery at least.

Slide the transducer caudad in small increments. You will observe the following: the portal vein extends to the left from the splenic vein, the hepatic artery disappears from the image or also swings left, and you can identify the origin of the celiac trunk at the aorta and its division into the hepatic and splenic arteries. In some cases you may see two sections of the hepatic artery in the same plane, as shown in Fig. 5.**8b**. This is explained by the curved course of the vessel, which loops out of the image plane and back in again. With luck, you can also identify the bile duct, which descends parallel to the vena cava.

As you continue to move the transducer caudally, the following occurs: you leave the portal vein and splenic vein behind, and a section of the superior mesenteric vein comes into view (Fig. 5.**8c**). Next to it is the section of the bile duct, just before it turns to the right toward the duodenum.

Fig. 5.8   **Defining the left portal vein branch in transverse sections**

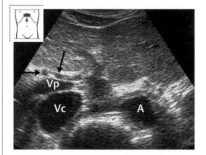 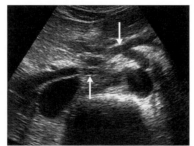 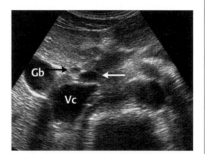

a High scan demonstrating the vena cava (Vc), aorta (A), portal vein (Vp), hepatic artery (↓), and bile duct (→).

b The transducer was moved to a slightly lower level. You see the junction of the portal vein with the splenic vein (↑). You also see the hepatic artery (↓) arising from the celiac trunk.

c The transducer was moved lower. The portal vein and hepatic artery have disappeared from the scan plane. You now see a section of the superior mesenteric vein (←) next to the bile duct (→). Gb = gallbladder, Vc = vena cava. This image corresponds to the diagram in Fig. 5.**7**.

Defining the porta hepatis in longitudinal sections

Figure 5.**9a** shows a longitudinal section through the porta hepatis. Though difficult to understand initially, this diagram is helpful in identifying the vessels with ultrasound.

Image the portal vein longitudinally as you did when identifying the bile duct (see p. 98). Identify the vena cava, portal vein, and bile duct. This scan should also show a cross section of the hepatic artery, even if it is somewhat difficult to identify (Fig. 5.**9b**). Move the transducer slightly to the left and observe how the bile duct elongates and runs downward toward the head of the pancreas (Fig. 5.**9c**). Also keep your eye on the hepatic artery, which moves very little on the screen because it first runs somewhat obliquely and then horizontally to the left toward the aorta. Move the transducer farther to the left. The hepatic artery continues to approach the aorta. The portal vein merges with the splenic vein, and the bile duct disappears from the image plane (Fig. 5.**9d**).

Fig. 5.9 *Defining the porta hepatis in longitudinal sections*

a Longitudinal section through the porta hepatis, corresponding to image ***b***. The plane of section passes through the vena cava (Vc), portal vein (Vp), hepatic artery (Ah), and bile duct (Dhc). L = liver, P = pancreas, S = stomach.
Notice that the hepatic artery, portal vein, and bile duct are anterior to the vena cava. The hepatic artery and bile duct course anterior to the portal vein. The hepatic artery is cranial to the bile duct. It impresses the bile duct posteriorly and the portal vein anteriorly.

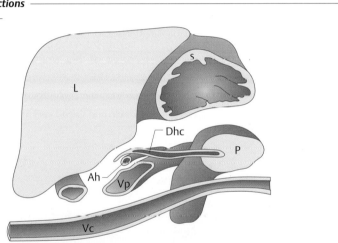

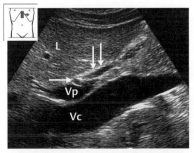

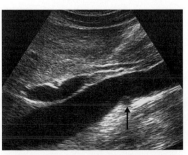

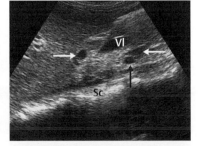

b Longitudinal scan through the porta hepatis. You see the portal vein (Vp) anterior to the vena cava (Vc). Anterior to the portal vein is the hepatic artery (→), which impresses the portal vein and bile duct (↓↓). L = liver.

c The transducer was moved slightly to the left. The bile duct has passed into the head of the pancreas. You also see the right renal artery (↑), which crosses under the vena cava.

d The transducer was moved farther to the left. You see the hepatic artery (→) and splenic vein (Vl). The bile duct is no longer in the image plane. You also see the left renal vein (←), which runs anterior to the right renal artery (↑). Sc = spinal column.

Organ Details: Details of the Vessels in the Porta Hepatis

Portal vein

The portal vein receives blood from the superior mesenteric vein, splenic vein, inferior mesenteric vein, and the coronary vein of the stomach. Generally the two latter veins cannot be identified. The portal vein is 6–8 cm long and up to 10–13 mm in diameter.

Defining the splenic vein and superior mesenteric vein in longitudinal sections

Take another look at Figs. 5.**1** and 5.**2**. Notice that the splenic vein and superior mesenteric vein are almost at right angles to each other, the splenic vein entering from the left and the superior mesenteric vein coming from below. Because of this arrangement, the vessels display typical sectional patterns in longitudinal and transverse scans (Figs. 5.**10**, 5.**11**).

Fig. 5.10 Defining the superior mesenteric vein and splenic vein in longitudinal sections

a Longitudinal section through the portal vein confluence (Vp) (plane 1, corresponds to image **b**). Medial to the confluence is the superior mesenteric vein (Vms) (plane 2, corresponds to image **c**), and farther medially is the splenic vein (Vl) (plane 3, corresponds to image **d**). L = liver, Lc = caudate lobe, Vc = vena cava.

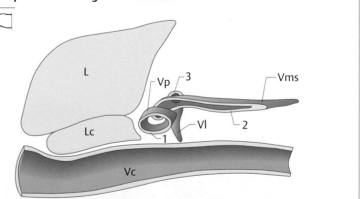

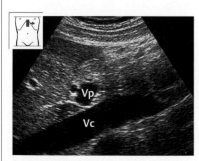

b Longitudinal scan over the vena cava (Vc) and portal vein (Vp).

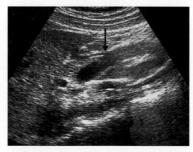

c The transducer was moved slightly to the left, almost out of the plane of the portal vein. The superior mesenteric vein (↓) is clearly defined.

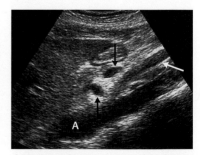

d The transducer was moved farther to the left, showing a cross section of the splenic vein (↓). The aorta (A) and superior mesenteric artery (←) are also seen. Splenic vein (↑).

Image the portal vein and vena cava in the familiar longitudinal scan (Fig. 5.**10 b**). Slowly move the transducer to the left. Observe how the section of the portal vein elongates to the superior mesenteric vein (Fig. 5.**10 c**). If you now move the transducer farther to the left, the longitudinal section of the superior mesenteric vein disappears from the image and the rounded section of the splenic vein comes into view (Fig. 5.**10 d**).

Defining the splenic vein and superior mesenteric vein in transverse sections

Demonstrate the vena cava and portal vein in an upper abdominal transverse scan (Fig. 5.**11 b**). Move the transducer caudad in small increments. Observe how the section of the portal vein at the confluence elongates to the left, becoming the splenic vein (Fig. 5.**11 c**). As the transducer is moved lower, the section of the splenic vein disappears from the image, and the cross section of the superior mesenteric vein comes into view (Fig. 5.**11 d**).

Fig. 5.11 Defining the splenic vein and superior mesenteric vein in transverse sections

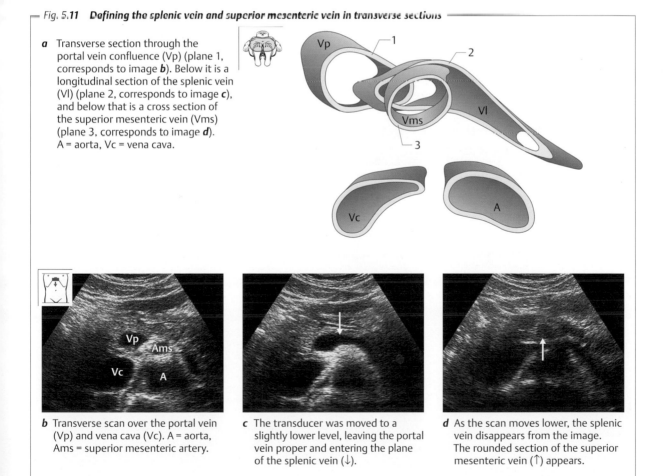

a Transverse section through the portal vein confluence (Vp) (plane 1, corresponds to image ***b***). Below it is a longitudinal section of the splenic vein (Vl) (plane 2, corresponds to image ***c***), and below that is a cross section of the superior mesenteric vein (Vms) (plane 3, corresponds to image ***d***). A = aorta, Vc = vena cava.

b Transverse scan over the portal vein (Vp) and vena cava (Vc). A = aorta, Ams = superior mesenteric artery.

c The transducer was moved to a slightly lower level, leaving the portal vein proper and entering the plane of the splenic vein (↓).

d As the scan moves lower, the splenic vein disappears from the image. The rounded section of the superior mesenteric vein (↑) appears.

Abnormalities of the portal vein

Portal vein dilatation. Dilatation of the portal vein (Fig. 5.**12**) is observed in portal hypertension. This can result from an intrahepatic obstruction (cirrhosis), prehepatic obstruction (portal vein thrombosis, see below), or posthepatic obstruction (Budd-Chiari syndrome, rare). The normal diameter of the portal vein is highly variable, however. A better way to check for elevated portal venous pressure is to assess the change of caliber with respiration. Normally the portal vein diameter increases on inspiration. Absence of this increase means that the pressure is elevated.

Portal vein thrombosis. Portal vein thrombosis is seen in patients with chronic liver diseases, pancreatic carcinoma, hematologic diseases, paraneoplastic syndromes, and other disorders. Ultrasound typically shows dilatation of the portal vein and an echogenic thrombus proximal to the affected site (Fig. 5.**13**).

Cavernous transformation. When portal vein thrombosis is of long standing, it can lead to partial recanalization with the development of paraportal collaterals and cavernous transformation of the portal vein (Fig. 5.**14**).

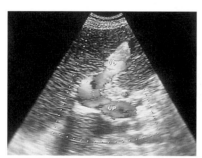

*Fig. 5.**12**   Dilatation of the portal vein in portal hypertension.*

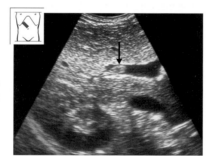

*Fig. 5.**13**   Portal vein thrombosis.* The portal vein is dilated proximal to the echogenic thrombus (↓).

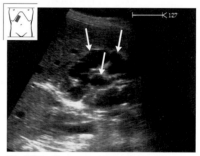

*Fig. 5.**14**   Cavernous transformation.* Tortuous veins in the region of the porta hepatis (↓).

Bile duct

The normal bile duct is 6 mm or less in diameter. A width greater than 9 mm is generally abnormal and indicates an obstruction. However, if the patient has had a cholecystectomy, the bile duct may be as large as 9 mm without signifying an outflow obstruction (Fig. 5.**15**).

Biliary obstruction (Figs. 5.**16**, 5.**17**). Impacted stones are the most frequent cause of common duct obstruction. In some cases the stones can be visualized with ultrasound. The prepapillary part of the bile duct is often difficult to define, however.

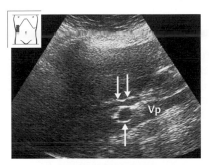

Fig. 5.15 Post-cholecystectomy.
Very large bile duct (↓↓), approximately 6 mm in diameter. Hepatic artery (↑). Vp = portal vein.

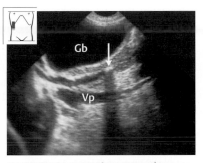

Fig. 5.16 Common duct stone (↓).
Gb = gallbladder, Vp = portal vein.

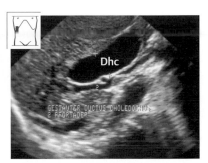

Fig. 5.17 Extreme dilatation of the bile duct in pancreatic carcinoma.

6 Gallbladder

Organ Boundaries

The gallbladder lies beneath the right costal arch, where it is covered mainly by the liver. Just caudal to it are the transverse colon and right colic flexure. These three structures — the liver, costal arch, and colon — form the anatomical framework within which the gallbladder is scanned. The liver is used as an acoustic window, while the colon and costal margin act as barriers. The acoustic windows that are available for scanning the gallbladder are relatively narrow (Figs. 6.**1**, 6.**2**).

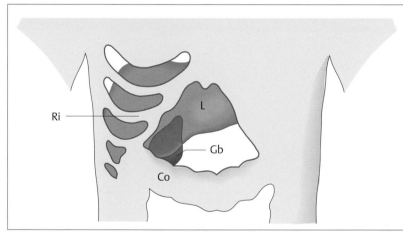

Fig. 6.**1** **Anterior approach to the gallbladder (Gb).** The colon (Co) and ribs (Ri) are barriers to scanning, while the liver (L) provides an acoustic window.

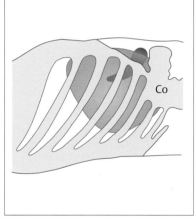

Fig. 6.**2** **Lateral approach to the gallbladder.** Again, the colon (Co) and costal arch are barriers while the liver provides an acoustic window.

Locating the gallbladder

Barriers to scanning

Every beginner has difficulty locating the gallbladder. Beside lack of experience, there are patient-related factors that can make the gallbladder difficult to find.
➤ The gallbladder has a small cross section.
➤ It may be hidden by bowel gas.
➤ It may be contracted.
➤ It lies behind the costal margin.

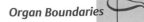

Optimizing the scanning conditions

The gallbladder is examined in the fasted patient. This includes abstinence from coffee and nicotine (which stimulate contraction). As in the liver, scanning conditions are improved by having the patient raise the right arm above the head. It is also helpful to scan at full inspiration.

Organ identification

KEY POINT

The sonographic characteristics of the gallbladder are: smooth margins, absence of internal echoes, and posterior acoustic enhancement.

Place the probe transversely on the right costal arch, approximately at the midclavicular line. Scan up into the liver at a steep angle (Fig. 6.3 b), then slowly angle the transducer downward. First you will see the portal vein (Fig. 6.3 c). Next the gallbladder will appear as an echo-free organ with smooth margins and posterior acoustic enhancement (Fig. 6.3 d). The longitudinal scan in Fig. 6.3 a indicates the position of the three transverse scans in the figure.

Fig. 6.**3** *Identifying the gallbladder*

a Upper abdominal longitudinal scan through the liver (L), portal vein (Vp), gallbladder (Gb), and vena cava (Vc). The planes of transverse scans **b–d** are indicated.

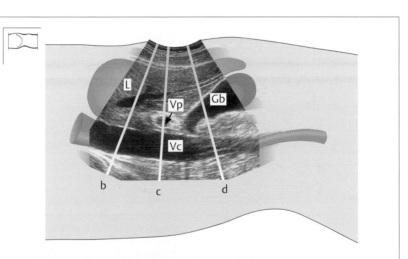

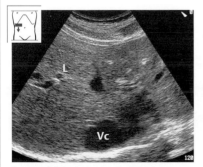

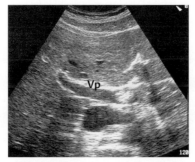

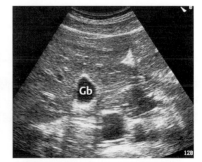

b Liver (L) and vena cava (Vc).

c The transducer was angled caudad: liver, vena cava, and portal vein (Vp).

d The transducer was angled lower, scanning through the gallbladder (Gb).

Imaging the entire gallbladder ———————————

You will learn below how to scan the entire gallbladder systematically using parallel upper abdominal transverse scans, upper abdominal longitudinal scans, and intercostal flank scans.

Defining the gallbladder in upper abdominal transverse scans

Image the gallbladder in an upper abdominal transverse scan, positioning it slightly to the left of the midline on the screen. Pause briefly, then scan all the way down the gallbladder in parallel transverse sections (Fig. 6.**4**).

— Fig. 6.**4**   *Defining the gallbladder in upper abdominal transverse scans* —————

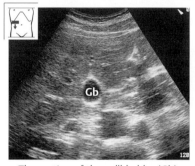

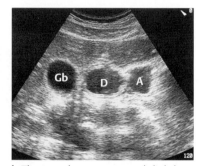

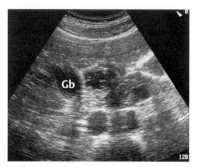

a The section of the gallbladder (Gb) is identified.

b The transducer was moved slightly lower. Next to the gallbladder are the duodenum (D) and the antrum of the stomach (A). A view of this quality is obtained only when the stomach and duodenum are filled with fluid. Compare the position of the gallbladder in scans *a* and *b*. It occupies the middle third of the image in *a* and is on the left side of the screen in *b*, indicating that the long axis of the gallbladder is directed somewhat laterally.

c The transducer was moved caudad and angled lower. The section of the gallbladder appears smaller again.

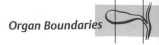

Defining the gallbladder in upper abdominal longitudinal scans

Obtain a transverse section of the gallbladder that displays its largest diameter. Then rotate the probe 90° while watching the screen. Observe how the rounded shape of the gallbladder assumes the elliptical shape of a longitudinal section (Fig. 6.**5a**). Move the transducer to the right in small increments until the gallbladder disappears (Fig. 6.**5b,c**). Scan from the right to the left side of the gallbladder.

*Fig. 6.***5** ***Defining the gallbladder in upper abdominal longitudinal scans***

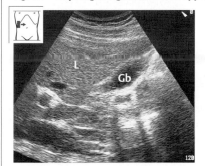

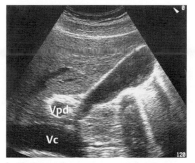

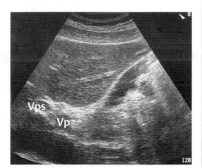

a Lateral longitudinal scan of the gallbladder (Gb). Observe its typical location on the visceral surface of the liver (L).

b The transducer was moved a short distance medially. You already know this section from Fig. 6.**3a**. It shows the liver and gallbladder along with a section of the right portal vein branch (Vpd) and the vena cava (Vc). The bright echoes behind the gallbladder are from gas in the duodenum.

c The transducer was moved farther medially. This scan cuts a smaller section of the gallbladder, and it cuts the main trunk of the portal vein (Vp). Just lateral and anterior to the venous trunk is the left portal vein branch (Vps).

Locating and defining the gallbladder with intercostal flank scans

The third scanning approach to the gallbladder is the lateral approach through the intercostal spaces. The intercostal approach can be challenging initially, but with proper technique it can provide excellent views of the gallbladder.

Place the transducer in a lower intercostal space at the midaxillary line. Direct the beam between the ribs, and define a caudal section of the liver. Sweep the scan from posterior to anterior in a fan-shaped pattern. If necessary, move the transducer to a more anterior intercostal space and repeat the scan. Figure 6.**6c** illustrates a typical intercostal view of the gallbladder.

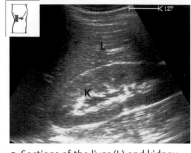

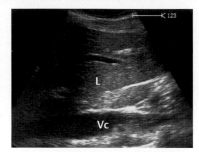

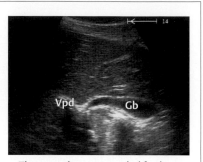

a Sections of the liver (L) and kidney (K).

b The scan plane was angled slightly anteriorly, demonstrating the liver and vena cava (Vc).

c The scan plane was angled farther anteriorly. The gallbladder (Gb) is now visible at the inferior border of the liver. The right portal vein branch (Vpd) is also seen.

The image in Fig. 6.**6 c** requires some explanation. The view obtained with an intercostal flank scan is somewhat similar to an upper abdominal longitudinal scan. Figure 6.**7** shows how the viewing angles differ.

Fig. 6.**7**   *Upper abdominal longitudinal scan of gallbladder, intercostal flank scan*

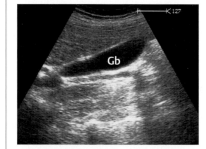

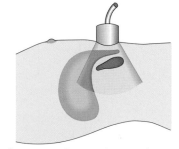

a Upper abdominal longitudinal scan of the gallbladder (Gb).

b Diagram showing the transducer placement for image *a*.

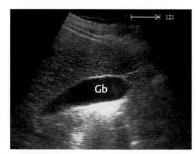

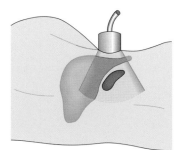

c Intercostal flank scan of the gallbladder.

d Transducer placement for the intercostal scan. The diagram shows the view from the posterior aspect.

Variable position of the gallbladder

In typical cases the long axis of the gallbladder is directed laterally downward at an oblique angle. But it may also follow the long axis of the body, and occasionally it runs somewhat medially (Fig. 6.**8**).

The fundus of the gallbladder is usually located anteriorly, lying directly upon the inferior border of the liver (Fig. 6.**9**). In other cases it is located deep beneath the liver.

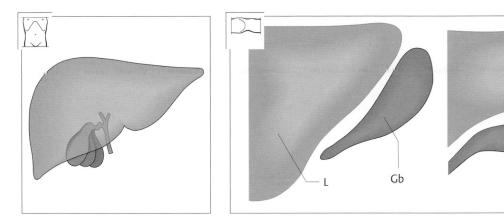

Fig. 6.8   Variable position of the gallbladder.

Fig. 6.9   Position of the gallbladder fundus in relation to the inferior hepatic border. L = liver, Gb = gallbladder.

Nonvisualization of the gallbladder

Table 6.**1**   Examiner-independent reasons for inability to find the gallbladder

Previous cholecystectomy
Obesity
Contracted gallbladder
Shrunken gallbladder
Stones filling the gallbladder
Echogenic gallbladder

There can be many reasons why the gallbladder is not seen with ultrasound. The most common reason for beginners is a simple lack of experience. The illustrations in this book were taken from cases with favorable scanning conditions, but the actual practice of gallbladder scanning can be more difficult. The most common examiner-independent causes of poor gallbladder visualization are listed in Table 6.**1**.

Prior cholecystectomy. Naturally, the gallbladder is not found in patients who have had a cholecystectomy. Elderly patients may have forgotten the operation, and subtle scars are easily overlooked in the dark examination room. You should specifically look for a cholecystectomy scar if the gallbladder is not found and the patient is unsure about his or her surgical history. If the organ has been removed, a very echogenic scar can usually be found in the gallbladder bed.

The series of images in Fig. 6.**10** illustrate a systematic search for the gallbladder or cholecystectomy scar, analogous to Fig. 6.**3**.

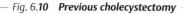

*Fig. 6.***10** ⎯ *Previous cholecystectomy*

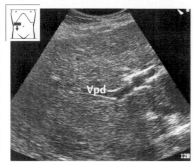

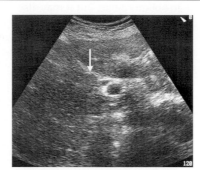

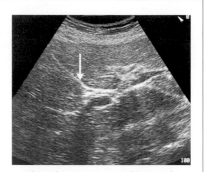

a Right portal vein branch (Vpd).

b Scan slightly below the level in *a* demonstrates a narrow band of high-level echoes (↑).

c When the scan is moved lower, the gallbladder should come into view. In its place, a fine, hyperechoic scar is seen (↓).

The width of a cholecystectomy scar is highly variable (Fig. 6.**11**).

Obesity. Marked obesity can make it very difficult to visualize the gallbladder in subcostal scans (Fig. 6.**12**). Limited views of the gallbladder can often be obtained in these cases with flank scans using the liver as an acoustic window.

Postprandial contraction. After meals the gallbladder may contract to the size of the portal vein lumen. When asking the patient whether he or she has eaten, remember that coffee or nicotine use can also cause the gallbladder to contract (Fig. 6.**13**).

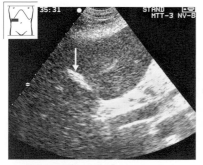

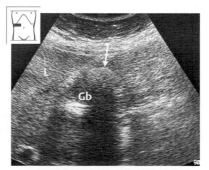

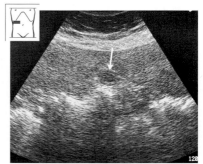

*Fig. 6.***11** ⎯ *Previous cholecystectomy.* Scan demonstrates a bright, rhomboid-shaped scar in the former gallbladder bed (↓).

*Fig. 6.***12** ⎯ *Obesity and gallstones.* The liver contours are indistinct, and the gallbladder wall is poorly demarcated from the outline of the liver (L). The gallbladder shows a small residual lumen with a stone (↓). Gb = gallbladder.

*Fig. 6.***13** ⎯ *Postprandial contraction of the gallbladder (↓).*

Shrunken gallbladder. The gallbladder may shrink from chronic inflammation. The bile becomes viscid and sludge or gallstones may form, causing loss of the fluid-filled lumen. It can be very difficult in these cases to delineate the gallbladder from the duodenum (Figs. 6.**14** – 6.**16**).

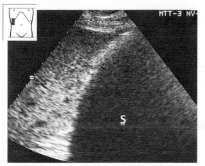

Fig. 6.14   Gallstones. The gallbladder is completely filled with stones, which cast a large, uniform acoustic shadow (S). The gallbladder lumen is not visualized.

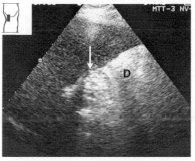

Fig. 6.15   Shrunken gallbladder. The gallbladder lumen is obliterated by small stones and debris (↓). The gallbladder is poorly delineated from the gas-filled duodenum (D).

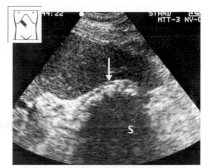

Fig. 6.16   Shrunken gallbladder. The gallbladder lumen is obliterated by stones and debris (↓), which cast a dense acoustic shadow (S).

Organ Details

LEARNING GOALS

➤ Identify the gallbladder regions in the sonogram.
➤ Determine the dimensions of the gallbladder.
➤ Evaluate the gallbladder wall.
➤ Evaluate the gallbladder contents.
➤ Recognize artifacts in gallbladder scanning.

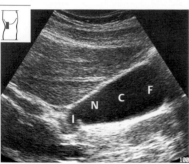

Fig. 6.17   Regions of the gallbladder.
F = fundus, Kp = body, Kl = neck,
I = infundibulum.

Regions of the gallbladder

The gallbladder consists of a fundus, body, neck, and infundibulum.

Sonographic identification of the gallbladder regions

Image the gallbladder in longitudinal section. Try to obtain an optimum view of the gallbladder regions in one image, and study that view (Fig. 6.**17**).

Size of the gallbladder

Reports of normal gallbladder size vary because the dimensions of the organ are highly variable. The gallbladder may be up to 12 cm in length. Most authors state a range of 9 – 11 cm for gallbladder length, with a transverse diameter up to 4 cm.

KEY POINTS

The normal gallbladder is 9 – 11 cm in length. The normal transverse width is 4 cm or less.

Gallbladder volume =
length × width × depth × 0.5 cm.

Sonographic determination of gallbladder size

The length and depth of the gallbladder are measured in an upper abdominal longitudinal scan, and the width is measured in a transverse scan. The volume of the gallbladder is then calculated using a simplified formula: length (cm) × width (cm) × depth (cm) × 0.5 (Fig. 6.**18**).

— Fig. 6.**18**   *Determining the dimensions of the gallbladder* —

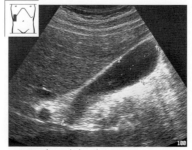 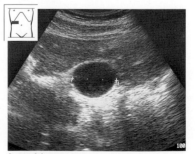

a Length and depth in upper
  abdominal longitudinal section.

b Width in transverse section.

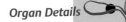

Enlargement of the gallbladder

Large gallbladders can occur as morphologic variants (Figs. 6.**19**, 6.**20**), especially in older patients and diabetics. Prolonged fasting also leads to a large gallbladder that may contain sludge.

If the transverse diameter of the gallbladder exceeds 4 cm, a pathologic condition should be suspected.

A normally distended gallbladder is distinguished from a hydropic gallbladder by its relatively lax appearance. In hydrops, the gallbladder is markedly distended due to an outflow obstruction, usually caused by a cystic or common duct stone (Fig. 6.**21**). The normal gallbladder is comparable to a water-filled balloon that is not under pressure, whereas the hydropic gallbladder is like a balloon that has been tightly inflated with an equal volume of air.

Table 6.**2** reviews the causes of a large gallbladder.

Table 6.**2** Causes of a large gallbladder

Morphologic variant

Fasting

Atony (diabetes mellitus)

Advanced age

Hydrops

Empyema

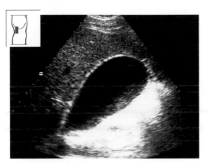

*Fig. 6.***19** *Healthy gallbladder.*
Transverse diameter of 4.7 cm in a fasted patient.

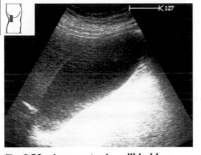

*Fig. 6.***20** *Large, atonic gallbladder* in a healthy female subject.

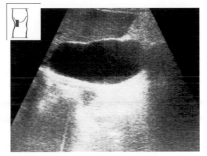

*Fig. 6.***21** *Gallbladder hydrops.*
The hydropic gallbladder is tightly distended and is tender to transducer pressure.

Variable shape of the gallbladder

The assessment of gallbladder shape is more useful than measuring its dimensions. With practice, you will gain an appreciation of the variability of normal gallbladder shapes. Frequently the gallbladder is pear-shaped (Fig. 6.**22 a**). It may also be round, elongated, or angulated (Fig. 6.**22 b,c**). The "Phrygian cap" gallbladder is one that is folded over at the fundus (Fig. 6.**22 d**). (A Phrygian cap is a tall, wedge-shaped cap whose crown is stuffed with material and folded forward.)

Fig. 6.22 **Gallbladder shapes**

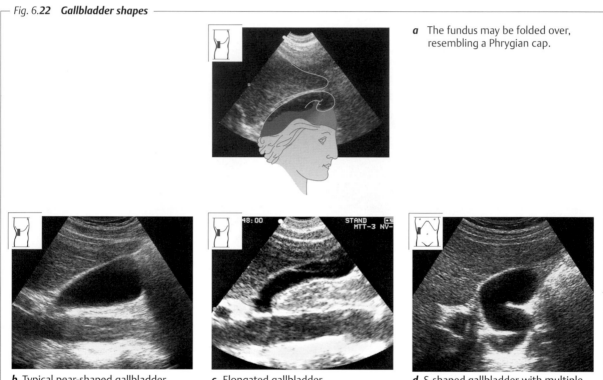

a The fundus may be folded over, resembling a Phrygian cap.

b Typical pear-shaped gallbladder.

c Elongated gallbladder.

d S-shaped gallbladder with multiple kinks.

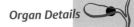

Gallbladder wall

The gallbladder wall consists of three layers: mucous, muscular, and serous. Under favorable conditions, these three layers can be identified with ultrasound, appearing as hyperechoic inner and outer layers and a less echogenic middle layer. This layered structure is most clearly appreciated in the partially contracted state (Fig. 6.**23**). However, the layers seen with ultrasound cannot be definitely assigned to the mural layers that can be distinguished histologically.

Sonographic assessment of the gallbladder wall

Wall thickness should be measured in the anterior wall of the gallbladder that lies against the posterior hepatic surface, as it can be difficult to delineate the posterior wall from the stomach or duodenum. The noncontracted gallbladder wall may be up to 4 mm thick (Fig. 6.**24**).

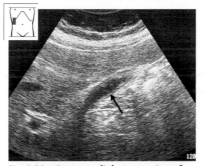

Fig. 6.**23** **Postprandial contraction of the gallbladder.** Ultrasound typically shows well-defined wall layers (↑) and a narrow lumen.

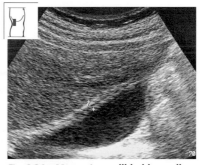

Fig. 6.**24** **Measuring gallbladder wall thickness (+ – +).** Intercostal flank scan of the gallbladder clearly demonstrates the three-layered structure: hyperechoic inner and outer layers with a hypoechoic middle layer.

Abnormalities of the gallbladder wall

Table 6.**3**   Causes of gallbladder wall thickening

Even the beginner can detect changes in wall thickness and echogenicity at an early stage (Figs. 6.**25** – 6.**31**). The possible causes of gallbladder wall thickening are listed in Table 6.**3**.

Contraction
Cholecystitis
Hepatic cirrhosis
Ascites
Acute viral hepatitis
Malignancy
Right-sided heart failure
Hypoproteinemia

Acute cholecystitis. Acute cholecystitis leads to hypoechoic mural thickening to more than 4 mm with irregular wall layers. It is also common to see a hypoechoic rim around the gallbladder bed (Figs. 6.**25**, 6.**26**).

Table 6.**4** lists the sonographic criteria of acute cholecystitis.

Table 6.**4** Sonographic features of acute cholecystitis

Tenderness to probe pressure

Thickened wall

Nonhomogeneous wall

Hypoechoic rim (halo)

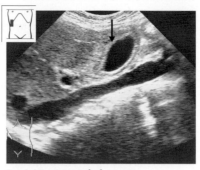

Fig. 6.25 **Acute cholecystitis.** The gallbladder wall is thickened and shows layers of different echogenicity (↓).

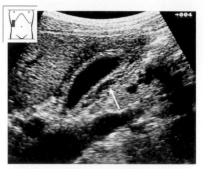

Fig. 6.26 **Acute cholecystitis.** Nonhomogeneous mural thickening, with areas of very low echogenicity (↑).

Chronic cholecystitis. Chronic cholecystitis often leads to nonhomogeneous, hyperechoic thickening of the gallbladder wall (Figs. 6.**27**, 6.**28**).

Table 6.**5** Sonographic features of chronic cholecystitis

Decreased size of the gallbladder

Mural thickening

Hyperechoic wall

Lack of contractility

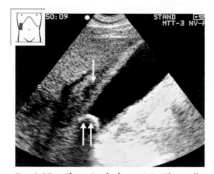

Fig. 6.27 **Chronic cholecystitis.** The gallbladder wall is thickened and hyperechoic. As in this case, a gallstone is usually present (↑↑). A hypoechoic streak is visible in the gallbladder bed (↓), signifying an acute exacerbation of the disease.

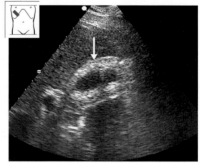

Fig. 6.28 **Chronic cholecystitis.** The gallbladder wall is markedly thickened and shows increased echogenicity (↓).

Porcelain gallbladder. This refers to calcification of the gallbladder wall as a result of chronic cholecystitis. Typically the whole gallbladder casts a more or less pronounced acoustic shadow. The posterior wall of the gallbladder is still well-defined, and the lumen contains faint internal echoes (Fig. 6.29).

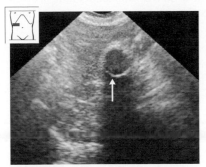

Fig. 6.29 Porcelain gallbladder. The calcified gallbladder wall appears as a thin ring (↑). Typical findings are a visible lumen and a bright posterior wall.

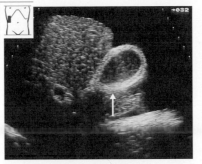

Fig. 6.30 Gallbladder in ascites. The gallbladder wall shows concentric thickening (↑) with smooth contours.

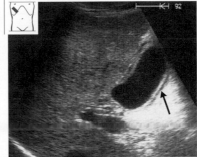

Fig. 6.31 Gallbladder in hepatic cirrhosis. The layers of the gallbladder wall appear markedly accentuated (↑).

Gallbladder contents

The healthy gallbladder is a fluid-filled hollow organ with no internal echoes.

Ultrasound appearance of the gallbladder contents

The sonographic hallmark of a healthy gallbladder is an almost echo-free lumen. It is not uncommon, however, to find internal echoes produced by artifacts (see p. 123).

Abnormal gallbladder contents

Table 6.**6** Sonographic features
of gallstones

Echogenicity

Posterior acoustic shadow

Mobility

Gallstone. Gallstones are among the most common pathologic findings in upper abdominal sonography. They vary greatly in size and number (Figs. 6.**32**–6.**34**). Their ultrasound appearance is highly variable, depending on the composition, shape, location, and size of the stones. The typical criteria for an ultrasound diagnosis are a stone echo in the echo-free gallbladder lumen, distal acoustic shadowing, and movement as the patient changes position (Table 6.**6**).

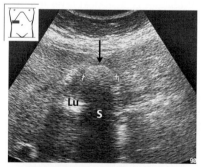

Fig. 6.32 Multiple gallstones. The individual stones (↑) cannot be clearly differentiated from one another. L = liver, Gb = gallbladder, S = acoustic shadows.

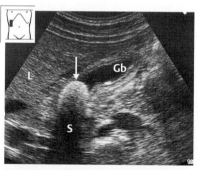

Fig. 6.33 Multiple gallstones (↑↑) on the posterior wall of the gallbladder.

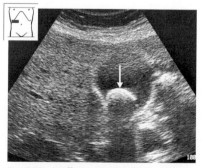

Fig. 6.34 Stone-filled gallbladder. This gallbladder is completely filled with stones (↓↓) and sludge. A residual lumen is no longer detectable.

The composition of a gallstone cannot be accurately inferred from its ultrasound appearance. Stones with a high cholesterol content have some degree of through-transmission and show an internal structure (Figs. 6.**35**, 6.**36**). A high calcium content produces a bright reflection on the insonated surface of the stone (Fig. 6.**37**).

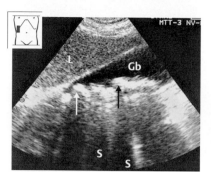

Fig. 6.35 Cholesterol-rich gallstone (↓) with a homogeneous internal structure. Small residual lumen. S = acoustic shadow, Lu = gas in the duodenum.

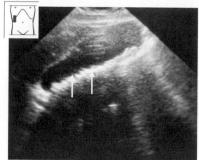

Fig. 6.36 Solitary stone in the gallbladder (↓). The cholesterol stone still exhibits internal structure. L = liver, Gb = gallbladder, S = acoustic shadow.

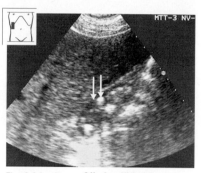

Fig. 6.37 Gallstone with a high calcium content, appearing as a sharp, crescent-shaped reflection (↓).

The most difficult gallstones to detect are infundibular stones and stones in a shrunken gallbladder (Figs. 6.**38** – 6.**40**, Table 6.**7**). Conversely, the infundibular region is often difficult to define and may exhibit phenomena that resemble the shadow cast by a stone (Table 6.**8**). Gas in the duodenum can also mimic a gallstone on cursory examination.

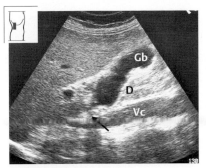

Fig. 6.38 **Infundibular stones.**
Small, shadowing calculi (↑) in the infundibulum are easy to miss.
Gb = gallbladder, D = duodenum, Vc = vena cava.

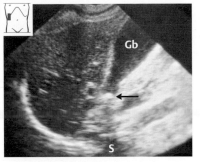

Fig. 6.39 **Infundibular stone (←).**
S = acoustic shadow, Gb = gallbladder.

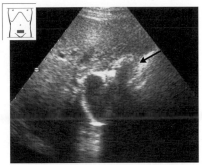

Fig. 6.40 **Gallstone in the folded fundus (←).**

Table 6.7 False-positive diagnosis of gallstones

Gas in the duodenum
Lateral cystic shadowing
Artifacts in the gallbladder neck
Polyps

Table 6.8 False-negative diagnosis of gallstones

Infundibular stones
Stone in a folded fundus

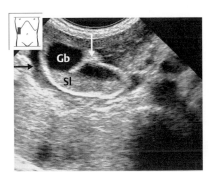

Fig. 6.41 **Sludge.** Sludge appears as an echogenic sediment on the floor of the folded (↓) gallbladder. Ascites (→) is also present. Sl = sludge, Gb = gallbladder.

Gallbladder sludge. Sludge is a collection of viscid bile that has settled on the gallbladder wall. It may occur after several days of fasting, especially in patients on parenteral nutrition. Ultrasound demonstrates the typical, smooth-bordered sediment, which contrasts with the overlying liquid bile (Fig. 6.**41**). The sonographic features and differential diagnosis of gallbladder sludge are reviewed in Tables 6.**9** and 6.**10**.

Table 6.9 Sonographic features of gallbladder sludge

Echogenic sediment
Bile–sludge level
Mobility

Table 6.10 Differential diagnosis of gallbladder sludge

Sand
Beam-width artifact
Empyema
Acute cholecystitis
Chronic cholecystitis

Echogenic bile. Sludge completely filling the gallbladder leads to the phenomenon of echogenic bile, in which a clear lumen is no longer seen (Fig. 6.**42**).

Gallbladder sand. A sediment with elements that cast an acoustic shadow is called biliary sand (Figs. 6.**43**, 6.**44**).

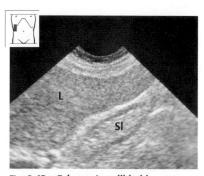

Fig. 6.42   Echogenic gallbladder.
The gallbladder is completely filled with echogenic sludge (Sl), which does not cast an acoustic shadow. L = liver.

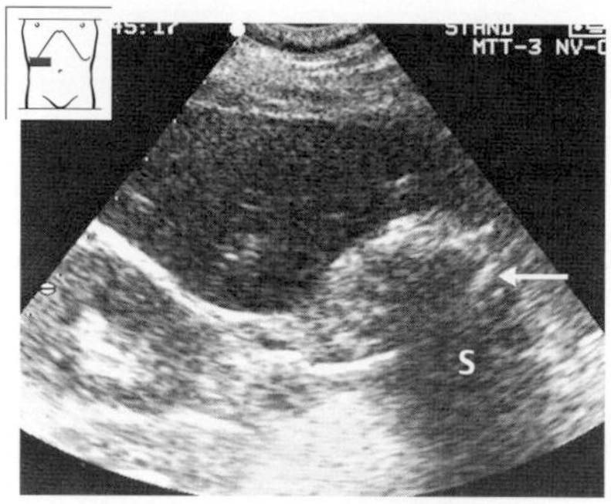

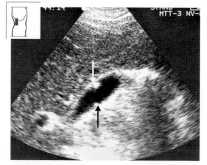

Fig. 6.43   Sand in the gallbladder.
Biliary sand (←) fills the gallbladder, producing a nonhomogeneous echo pattern and a posterior acoustic shadow (S).
L = liver, K = kidney.

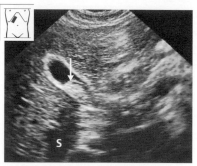

Fig. 6.44   Sand in the gallbladder.
Nonhomogeneous, echogenic sediment (↓) on the gallbladder floor, with an associated acoustic shadow (S).

Polypoid lesions

It is not unusual to find circumscribed polypoid lesions attached to the gallbladder wall. Since they require differentiation from gallstones, they are included here under the heading of "gallbladder contents."

Cholesterol polyps. These are hemispherical, highly reflective masses of cholesterol deposits, a few millimeters in size, that project into the gallbladder lumen (Figs. 6.**45**, 6.**46**). They do not cast an acoustic shadow.

KEY POINT

Unlike gallstones, gallbladder polyps are not mobile and do not cast an acoustic shadow.

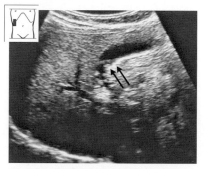

Fig. 6.45   Cholesterol polyps (↑↑).
Hyperechoic nodules project into the gallbladder lumen and do not cast acoustic shadows.

Fig. 6.46   Multiple cholesterol polyps (↑↑). The polyps appear as broad-based lesions with irregular margins.

Gallbladder adenomas and carcinomas. Gallbladder adenomas are rare. Most appear as relatively large protrusions (> 5 mm) of moderate echogenicity with smooth or irregular margins (Figs. 6.**47**, 6.**48**). Large adenomas (> 10 mm) cannot be positively distinguished from carcinomas (Fig. 6.**49**) and should be treated operatively.

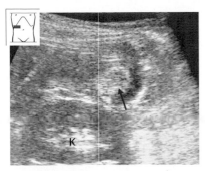

*Fig. 6.**47** Gallbladder adenoma (↑).*
A mass with relatively smooth margins and a nonhomogeneous echo pattern occupies most of the gallbladder lumen. N = kidney.

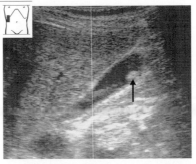

*Fig. 6.**48** Gallbladder adenoma.*
Scan shows a small globular mass projecting into the gallbladder lumen (↑). The lesion is roughly isoechoic to the gallbladder wall.

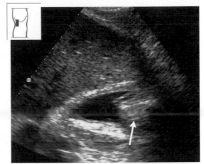

*Fig. 6.**49** Gallbladder carcinoma (↑).*
The fundus is occupied by a large mass arising from the wall.

Special acoustic phenomena in gallbladder scanning

Table 6.**11** Acoustic phenomena that can be confusing in gallbladder examinations

Posterior acoustic enhancement

Lateral cystic shadowing

Beam-width artifacts

Resonance artifacts

Gas in the duodenum

In scanning the gallbladder, you should be aware of several acoustic phenomena that may become a source of confusion (Table 6.**11**).

Lateral edge shadows. Shadows extending from the lateral edges of the gallbladder (see p. 18) can mimic the shadows cast by gallstones (Fig. 6.**50**).

Beam-width artifact. Beam-width artifacts (see p. 15) may be mistaken for sludge (Fig. 6.**51**).

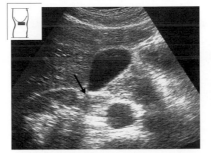

*Fig. 6.**50** Edge shadows (↓).*

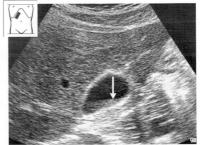

*Fig. 6.**51** Beam-width artifact (↓), appearing as a layer of fine echoes on the posterior gallbladder wall.*

Artifacts in the area of the gallbladder neck. The gallbladder neck can be very difficult to image clearly. Stones in this area may be overlooked (Fig. 6.**38**), and shadowing effects can mimic the presence of stones (Fig. 6.**52**).

Gas in the duodenum. The proximity of the duodenum to the gallbladder can sometimes produce surprising effects. Gas can simulate a stone (Fig. 6.**53**), and a food bolus can mimic neoplastic wall thickening (Fig. 6.**54**). The observation of duodenal peristalsis suggests the correct diagnosis, however.

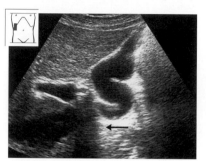

Fig. 6.*52   Acoustic shadow (←)*
behind the gallbladder neck.

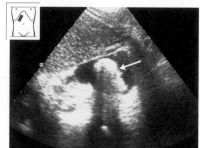

Fig. 6.**53   Gas in the duodenum (←)**
with acoustic shadowing. Part of the
duodenum bulges into the gallbladder
during a peristaltic contraction and casts
a posterior acoustic shadow.

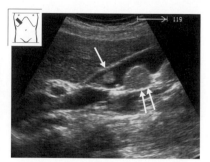

Fig. 6.**54   Food bolus in the duodenum**
and a gallbladder polyp. The duodenum bulges into the gallbladder from
behind, creating the impression of a
spherical mass on the gallbladder wall
(↑↑). There is also a pedunculated
polyp in the gallbladder neck (↓).

Anatomical Relationships

LEARNING GOALS

➤ Identify the gallbladder regions in the sonogram.

In examining the gallbladder, you have already noticed, regardless of what scanning approach you use (transverse subcostal, longitudinal, or intercostal), that the image area in the lower right-hand part of the monitor appears chaotic while the area at upper left is dominated by the orderly structure of the liver (Figs. 6.**55**, 6.**56**).

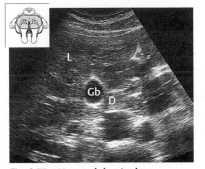

Fig. 6.55 **Upper abdominal transverse scan of the gallbladder.** The homogeneous texture of the liver (L) is visible at upper left. The gallbladder (Gb) is at the center of the image, and gas-filled bowel loops (D) produce a chaotic echo pattern at lower right.

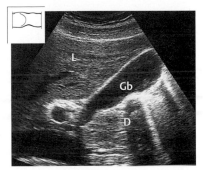

Fig. 6.56 **Upper abdominal longitudinal scan of the gallbladder.** The same general pattern is seen in the longitudinal plane: homogeneous echoes from the liver (L) at upper left, the gallbladder (Gb) at the center, and chaotic echoes from gas-filled bowel loops (D) at lower right.

Picture where this chaos is located in relation to the gallbladder. Its location in the lower right part of the image means that it is inferior, posterior, and medial to the gallbladder. It is caused by the gas-containing organs that border the gallbladder on three sides: the antrum and duodenal bulb (medially), the second part of the duodenum (inferomedially), and the colic flexure (inferiorly). The head of the pancreas, which is enclosed by the duodenal loop, is medial to the gallbladder. The gallbladder is related superiorly, anteriorly, and laterally to the liver (Figs. 6.**57**, 6.**58**). Despite the variability in shape, size, and position of the gallbladder, these relationships are observed consistently. They will be explored below.

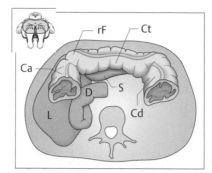

*Fig. 6.**57***   ***View into the abdomen from below,*** showing the ascending colon (Ca), transverse colon (Ct), descending colon (Cd), duodenum (D), gastric antrum (M), and liver (L). The gallbladder is hidden by the right flexure (rF).

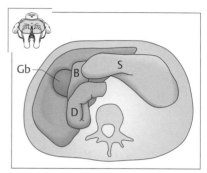

*Fig. 6.**58***   ***Same view as in Fig. 6.57.*** The colon has been removed to expose the gallbladder (Gb), which lies on the inferior surface of the liver and is framed by the antrum (M), duodenal bulb (B), and duodenum (D).

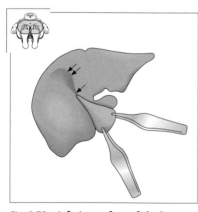

*Fig. 6.**59***   ***Inferior surface of the liver viewed from below.*** The gallbladder has been mobilized and reflected from its bed. Notice that the gallbladder bed forms a rounded depression at the level of the fundus (←←) and tapers to a sharp angle at the gallbladder neck (←).

Relationship of the gallbladder to the liver

You have already learned about this relationship when you used the liver as an acoustic window for scanning the gallbladder. Now you will define this relationship in somewhat greater detail. The gallbladder is nestled in a depression on the inferior surface of the liver. The depth of this depression is highly variable, but its shape shows some degree of consistency. The roof of the depression changes its shape from below upward. While it forms a smooth semicircle inferiorly at the level of the gallbladder fundus, it forms an acute angle superiorly at the level of the gallbladder neck (Fig. 6.**59**). In the roof of this depression, the gallbladder fossa, the gallbladder is attached to the undersurface of the liver. This site is easily recognized as a deep groove in an anatomical section, whereas in the gross anatomy of the liver surface it is considered equivalent to the gallbladder bed. As a result, it is often unfamiliar to the beginner. It can usually be identified sonographically as the interlobar fissure.

Defining the interlobar fissure

Place the probe transversely at the level of the midclavicular line and image the gallbladder as previously described. Angle the transducer cephalad, and observe how the cross section of the gallbladder dwindles in size. The moment it disappears, the interlobar fissure will appear in its place as a narrow or occasionally thick band (Figs. 6.**60**, 6.**61**). Often this fissure can be defined even more clearly by rotating the transducer to a subcostal oblique scan parallel to the costal margin.

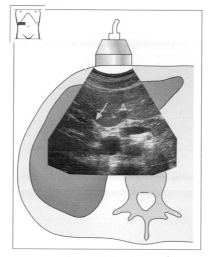

*Fig. 6.**60*** **The interlobar fissure (↓).**

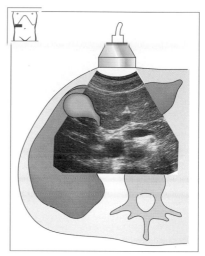

*Fig. 6.**61*** **Same scan as in Fig. 6.60.** The gallbladder has been drawn into the image, showing its location in front of the scan plane. The cranial extent of the interlobar fissure is variable. Watch the band disappear when you angle the scan higher. It is an anatomic landmark that you can use to positively identify the gallbladder itself or the gallbladder bed following cholecystectomy.

Defining the gallbladder bed

The interlobar fissure is the ridge atop the gallbladder bed. The roof is formed by the hepatic parenchyma. Image the gallbladder again in transverse section. Angle the scan upward, and identify the interlobar fissure (Fig. 6.**62a**). Then scan down the length of the gallbladder and observe the changing shape of the gallbladder bed (Fig. 6.**62 b, c**).

Fig. 6.62 Defining the gallbladder bed

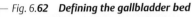
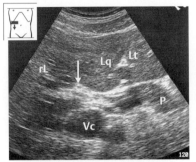
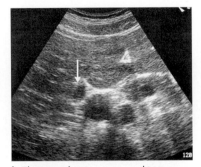
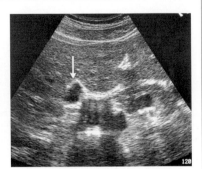

a Upper abdominal transverse scan immediately above the gallbladder. You see the sharp angle marking the start of the interlobar fissure (↓), also the right lobe of the liver (rL), the quadrate lobe (Lq), the ligamentum teres (Lt), the vena cava (Vc), and the pancreas (P).

b The transducer was moved to a slightly lower plane. The gallbladder neck (↓) can be seen.

c The transducer was moved lower. The gallbladder (↓) can be clearly identified, nestled in the concavity of the gallbladder bed.

Relationship of the gallbladder to the portal vein —

The portal vein and its branches are consistently seen when the gallbladder is examined. The spatial relationship of these structures will be detailed below (Figs. 6.**63** – 6.**65**). The gallbladder extends upward to the porta hepatis from below and to the right. At this level the gallbladder neck is related to the right portal vein branch.

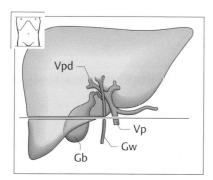

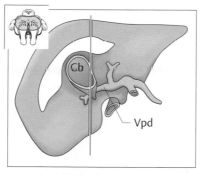

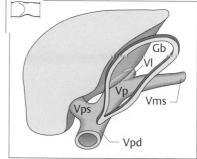

*Fig. 6.**63*** ***Frontal view.*** The liver, gall-bladder (Gb), bile duct (Gw), and portal vein (Vp) as they appear in textbooks of anatomy. Notice that the gallbladder neck lies just below the right portal vein branch (Vpd). The horizontal line indicates the plane of the transverse section in Fig. 6.***64***.

*Fig. 6.**64*** ***View of the porta hepatis in an upper abdominal transverse section.*** Notice that the gallbladder (Gb) lies directly below the right portal vein branch (Vpd). The vertical line indicates the plane of the longitudinal section in Fig. 6.***65***. Figure 6.***66 c*** shows the corresponding sonogram.

*Fig. 6.**65*** ***View of the porta hepatis in upper abdominal longitudinal section.*** Notice that the gallbladder neck almost touches the right portal vein branch (Vpd) from below. The gallbladder itself is shown only in outline for clarity. Behind (medial to) the gallbladder is the trunk of the portal vein (Vp), the terminal portions of the superior mesenteric vein (Vms) and splenic vein (Vl), and the left portal vein branch (Vps). Figure 6.***67 a*** shows the corresponding sonogram.

**Demonstrating the relationship of the gallbladder
to the portal vein in transverse section**

Place the probe transversely at about the level of the midclavicular line and
locate the vena cava. Center it on the screen, and scan upward into the liver.
Scan down the liver as you did for locating the gallbladder. Identify the porta
hepatis. Pause there a moment and take note of its position. You have defined
the region of the portal vein with the origin of the right main branch
(Fig. 6.**66a**). The gallbladder neck lies in front of the image plane and above
center, i.e., anterior. Scan slightly lower and define the cross section of the
gallbladder. Picture it extending from below upward, almost reaching the
right portal vein branch (Fig. 6.**66b, c**).

Fig. 6.66   **Demonstrating the relationship of the gallbladder to the portal vein in transverse sections**

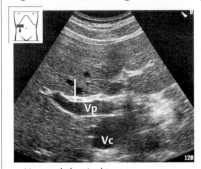

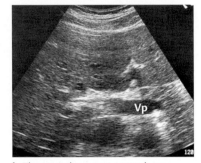

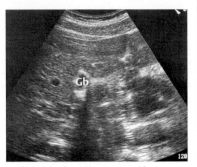

a Upper abdominal transverse scan
demonstrates the portal vein (Vp)
and its right main branch (↓).
Vc = vena cava.

b The transducer was moved very
slightly to a more caudal level. You
see the trunk of the portal vein (Vp),
whose right main branch is now
behind the plane of the scan.

c The transducer was moved lower.
The gallbladder neck (Gb) appears,
indicating its location just caudal to
the right portal vein branch.

Demonstrating the relationship of the gallbladder to the portal vein in longitudinal section

Position the transducer for an upper abdominal longitudinal scan, and look for the vena cava at the inferior border of the liver. Identify the portal vein confluence between the vena cava and inferior hepatic border. Slide the transducer to the right in small, parallel steps and observe the gallbladder appear in longitudinal section. Cranial to the gallbladder neck is a round vascular cross section. This is the right portal vein branch. Take note of its appearance, as it is a useful landmark. If you now slide the transducer farther to the right, you will see the section of the gallbladder moving upward and to the right, i.e., inferiorly, anteriorly, and laterally. The section of the portal vein moves upward and to the left, i.e., superiorly, anteriorly, and laterally. Now scan across the gallbladder and right portal vein from right to left, proceeding in small steps (Fig. 6.**67**).

*Fig. 6.**67*** *Demonstrating the relationship of the gallbladder to the portal vein in longitudinal sections*

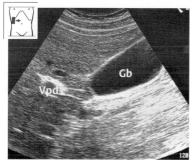 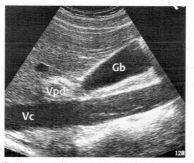 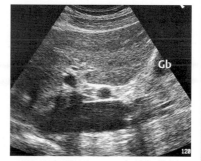

a Longitudinal scan through the gallbladder fundus (Gb) and right portal vein branch (Vpd). Notice the gap between the two structures.

b The transducer was moved very slightly to the left. The gallbladder neck (Gb) is now markedly closer to the right portal vein (Vpd). A longitudinal section of the vena cava (Vc) also appears.

c The transducer was moved farther to the left. Only a small section of the gallbladder fundus (Gb) is still visible at this level.

Relationship of the gallbladder to the antrum, bulb, and duodenum

The gallbladder extends laterally downward and slightly forward past the duodenum (Figs. 6.**68**–6.**70**). The frontal view of this topographic relationship is well known from textbooks of anatomy (Fig. 6.**68**), but it can be somewhat difficult to define with ultrasound because of gas in the duodenum.

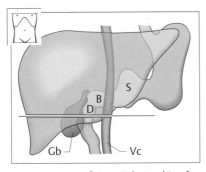

*Fig. 6.**68**   **Frontal view.*** Relationship of the gallbladder (Gb) to the duodenum (D), duodenal bulb (B), and gastric antrum (S). The line indicates the plane of the transverse section of this region in Fig. 6.**69**.

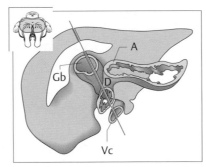

*Fig. 6.**69**   **Upper abdominal transverse section through the body of the gallbladder (Gb) and the duodenum (D).*** A = antrum, Vc = vena cava. Notice that the gallbladder passes laterally and anteriorly over the duodenum in a gentle arc. The line indicates the plane of the longitudinal section in Fig. 6.**70**. Important: The longitudinal section should cut both the gallbladder and the vena cava. When this is accomplished, the duodenum is always located between them. Compare this diagram with the image in Fig. 6.**71 c**.

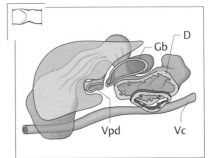

*Fig. 6.**70**   **Upper abdominal longitudinal section through the gallbladder (Gb) and vena cava (Vc).*** The duodenum (D) lies between them. The scan cuts the right portal vein branch (Vpd) at the bifurcation of the portal trunk. A lateral section of the duodenum has been drawn in front of the image plane to show that the duodenum may extend relatively far laterally. Compare this diagram with the image in Fig. 6.**72 c**.

Relationship to the antrum and first and second parts of the duodenum in transverse section

Place the probe transversely at about the level of the midclavicular line, and define the gallbladder in cross section. Identify the vena cava. You know that the second part of the duodenum lies between the gallbladder and vena cava. Angle the transducer up and down over the gallbladder and vena cava and look for the nonhomogeneous pattern of the duodenum (Fig. 6.**71**).

Fig. 6.71   *Demonstrating the relationship of the gallbladder to the duodenum in transverse sections*

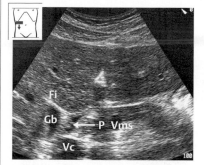 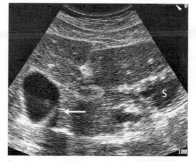 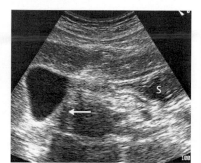

a Transverse scan demonstrates the gallbladder (Gb) and the interlobar fissure (Fi) at the interior border of the liver. Just medial to the gallbladder is a section of the duodenum (←). Vc = vena cava, P = pancreas, Vms = superior mesenteric vein.

b The transducer was moved slightly caudad. You see a section of the gallbladder and, just medial to it, the mixed echo pattern of the duodenum (←). The antrum of the stomach (S) is also seen at this level.

c The transducer was moved lower. The duodenum is poorly visualized (←), but the gastric antrum (S) is clearly displayed. Compare this image with Fig. 6.**69**.

Relationship to the antrum and first and second parts of the duodenum in longitudinal section

Place the probe longitudinally at about the level of the midclavicular line, and define the largest possible section of the gallbladder. Angle the probe until you have displayed the gallbladder and vena cava in one plane. This can be somewhat difficult initially but will become easier with practice. This plane serves as a sonographic landmark. Now move the transducer to the right in small, parallel steps until the section of the gallbladder disappears from the image. Then scan across the gallbladder and duodenum from right to left in small steps (Fig. 6.**72**).

---

*Fig. 6.**72*** ***Demonstrating the relationship of the gallbladder to the duodenum in longitudinal sections***

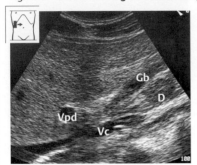 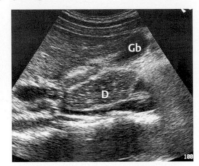 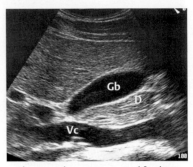

a You can just see the section of the gallbladder (Gb) and that of the vena cava (Vc). The duodenum (D) is interposed between them. Vpd = right portal vein branch.

b The transducer was moved slightly medially, displaying a larger section of the gallbladder (Gb). The duodenum (D) is clearly visualized.

c The transducer was moved farther medially. From anterior to posterior, you clearly see the gallbladder (Gb), duodenum (D), and vena cava (Vc). Compare this image with Fig. 6.**70**.

7 Pancreas

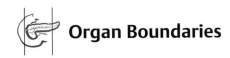 **Organ Boundaries**

> ➤ Locate and identify the pancreas.
> ➤ Demonstrate the entire pancreas.

The pancreas is located in the retroperitoneum, bounded on each side by the duodenum and the spleen. It lies transversely in the epigastrium, its axis directed at a slight angle from lower right to upper left.

Locating the pancreas

Barriers to scanning

The pancreas is often difficult to locate because of its posterior position. The main barrier to scanning the pancreas is gas in the stomach and bowel (Fig. 7.1).

Optimizing the scanning conditions

The pancreas, like the gallbladder, is best examined in the fasted patient. In some cases, visualization can be significantly improved by giving the patient an antigas medication. You can also apply local transducer pressure to push the gas aside. Of course, this should be done only after the other organs have been examined. Vision can be substantially improved by filling the stomach with water (500 ml, taken through a straw) (Fig. 7.2).

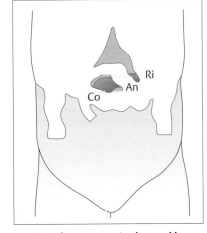

*Fig. 7.1 **The pancreas is obscured by the colon (Co), antrum (An), and costal arch (Ri).***

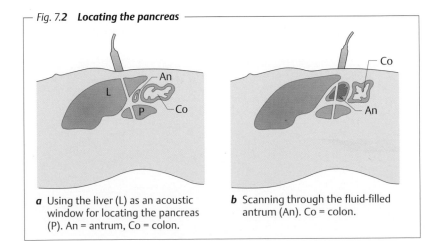

─ *Fig. 7.2 **Locating the pancreas*** ─

a Using the liver (L) as an acoustic window for locating the pancreas (P). An = antrum, Co = colon.

b Scanning through the fluid-filled antrum (An). Co = colon.

Organ identification

More than with other upper abdominal organs, identification of the pancreas relies on the use of landmarks. Your principal landmarks are the aorta and the splenic vein (Figs. 7.**3** – 7.**5**).

Position the transducer for a high upper abdominal transverse scan, and angle the scan slightly upward into the liver. Identify the aorta and vena cava. Now move the scan plane caudally in small increments. In some cases you will have to repeat this pass several times and use both sliding and angling movements of the probe to scan around gas in the stomach and bowel. As you scan down the aorta, look for the landmarks shown in Figs. 7.**3** and 7.**4**.

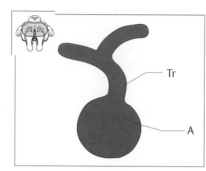

Fig. 7.**3**   *Aorta (A) and celiac trunk (Tr).* When you see this pattern in the transverse scan, you will find the pancreas at a slightly more caudal level.

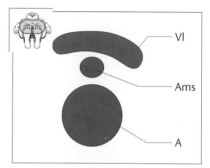

Fig. 7.**4**   *Aorta (A) plus a transverse section of the superior mesenteric artery (Ams) and a longitudinal section of the splenic vein (Vl).* When you see this pattern, you will almost always have the pancreas on the monitor. It appears as a gently curved structure passing anterior to the splenic vein. The ability to define the pancreas and delineate it from its surroundings will vary greatly from case to case.

Fig. 7.5 Locating the pancreas

a Upper abdominal longitudinal scan. The lines indicate the scan planes that are used in locating the pancreas. A = aorta, Tr = celiac trunk, Ams = superior mesenteric artery, P = pancreas, S = stomach, splenic vein (↑).

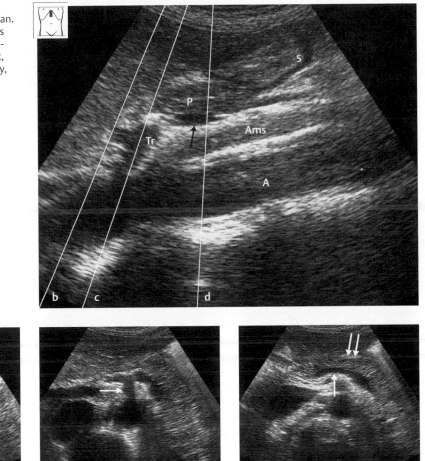

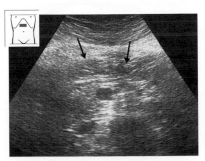

b Demonstrate the aorta (A).

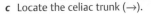

c Locate the celiac trunk (→).

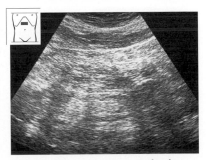

d Identify the splenic vein (↑) and the pancreas anterior to it (↓↓).

Difficulties in identifying the pancreas

The series of images shown above were obtained under ideal scanning conditions. In most examinations, however, the conditions will be less than ideal and often the pancreas cannot be completely visualized (Figs. **7.6** – 7.**8**).

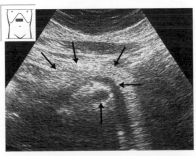

Fig. 7.**6** **Poor visualization of the pancreas (↓) due to obesity and overlying gas.**

Fig. 7.**7** **Obesity and pancreatic lipomatosis.** The superior mesenteric artery (↑) and splenic vein (←) are plainly seen, but the pancreas (↓↓↓) is poorly delineated.

Fig. 7.8 **The pancreas is completely obscured by gas.**

Imaging the entire pancreas

Below you will learn a systematic method of imaging the pancreas using parallel upper abdominal transverse and longitudinal scans. The tail of the pancreas can also be visualized by scanning through the spleen. This approach is described further under Anatomical Relationships (p. 150).

Defining the pancreas in upper abdominal transverse scans

Due to the length of the pancreas, several passes are needed to survey the entire organ in transverse sections (Figs. 7.**9**, 7.**10**).

Obtain a longitudinal section of the pancreas anterior to the splenic vein (Figs. 7.**9 b**, 7.**10 b**). Notice the gently curved shape of the pancreas above the landmark. Sweep through this section several times.

Then slide the transducer toward the tail of the pancreas, i.e., upward and to the left (Figs. 7.**9 c**, 7.**10 c**). Observe how the shape of the pancreas changes. You will notice that vision becomes poorer as the scan moves to the left. Scan through the tail of the pancreas. Its shape is highly variable.

Now return to the starting point, and move the transducer to the right toward the head of the pancreas (Figs. 7.**9 d**, 7.**10 a**). Again, observe the change in shape. Sweep through the head of the pancreas several times. While the body and tail of the pancreas have a relatively smooth, elliptical shape in the transverse scan, the contour of the head shows irregular depressions at several sites.

KEY POINTS

Multiple transverse and longitudinal scans are needed to survey the pancreas because of its length (approximately 15 cm).

The tail of the pancreas can be scanned through the spleen.

The splenic vein is the landmark for locating the pancreas in the transverse scan.

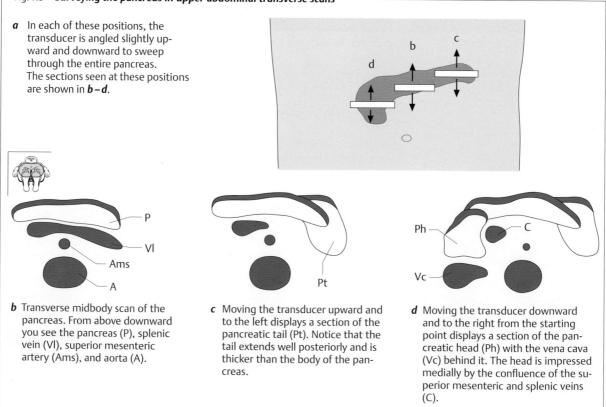

Fig. 7.**9** *Surveying the pancreas in upper abdominal transverse scans*

a In each of these positions, the transducer is angled slightly upward and downward to sweep through the entire pancreas. The sections seen at these positions are shown in **b–d**.

b Transverse midbody scan of the pancreas. From above downward you see the pancreas (P), splenic vein (Vl), superior mesenteric artery (Ams), and aorta (A).

c Moving the transducer upward and to the left displays a section of the pancreatic tail (Pt). Notice that the tail extends well posteriorly and is thicker than the body of the pancreas.

d Moving the transducer downward and to the right from the starting point displays a section of the pancreatic head (Ph) with the vena cava (Vc) behind it. The head is impressed medially by the confluence of the superior mesenteric and splenic veins (C).

Fig. 7.10   **Defining the pancreas in upper abdominal transverse scans**

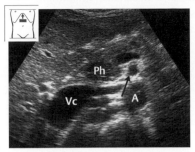

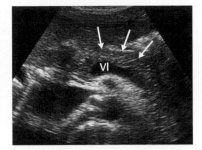

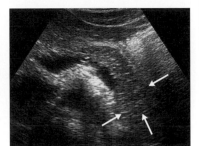

a Typical appearance of the pancreatic head (Ph) above the vena cava (Vc). A = aorta, superior mesenteric artery (↑).

b The transducer was moved slightly left to the midabdomen. You see the slender body of the pancreas (↓↓↓) lying anterior to the splenic vein (VI).

c The transducer was moved farther cephalad and to the left. You see the tail of the pancreas with its marked posterior extension (←↑→).

Defining the pancreas in upper abdominal longitudinal scans

KEY POINT

The aorta, celiac trunk, superior mesenteric artery, and splenic vein are the landmarks for identifying the pancreas in the longitudinal scan.

Start with the probe placed transversely on the upper abdomen, and define the body of the pancreas. While watching the screen, rotate the transducer to a longitudinal scan over the epigastrium. Keep the section of the pancreas in view, and angle the transducer slightly to locate the aorta. It will provide an aid to orientation. The key landmarks for locating the pancreas in the upper abdominal longitudinal scan are the aorta, celiac trunk, superior mesenteric artery, and splenic vein (Fig. 7.**11 a**).

Concentrate on the pancreas. Scanned longitudinally, the pancreas presents a flat, oblong cross section. Move the transducer to the left in parallel steps. As you saw before, vision is increasingly degraded by gas as you scan into the left upper abdomen. Nevertheless, try to make out the shape of the pancreatic tail. As you noticed in the previous series of upper abdominal transverse scans (which gave longitudinal views of the pancreas), the thickness of the organ increases in the tail region (Fig. 7.**11 b**).

Now return to the aorta and scan past it toward the right side. Notice that, while the portion of the pancreas over the aorta is flat but is still broad craniocaudally, as you move to the right the cross section of the pancreas thickens considerably, showing that you have reached the head (Fig. 7.**11 c**).

Fig. 7.11   **Surveying the pancreas in upper abdominal longitudinal scans**

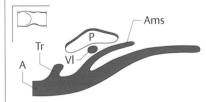

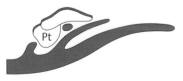

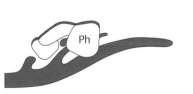

a Longitudinal landmarks for the pancreas (P) are the aorta (A), celiac trunk (Tr), superior mesenteric artery (Ams), and splenic vein (VI).

b Moving to the left displays a section of the pancreatic tail (Pt).

c Moving right displays a section of the pancreatic head (Ph).

Repeat this tail-to-head pass several times. Gain a clear spatial impression of the anatomy and location of the pancreas by observing how its cross section changes with transducer position (Fig. 7.**12**).

Fig. 7.12 Defining the pancreas in upper abdominal longitudinal scans

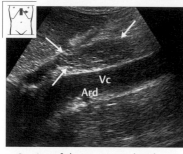

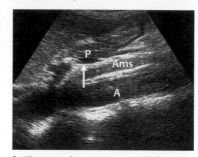

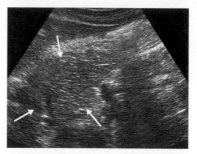

a Section of the pancreatic head (→↑←) anterior to the vena cava (Vc). Ard = right renal artery.

b The transducer was moved left to the upper midabdomen, displaying a section of the pancreas (P) with its landmarks, the aorta (A), superior mesenteric artery (Ams), and splenic vein (↑). Note the craniocaudal extent of the pancreas.

c The transducer was moved farther to the left. The thick tail of the pancreas (→↑←) is appreciated at this level.

Scanning the tail of the pancreas through the spleen

This approach is described fully in the section on Anatomical Relationships (p. 150).

Variable shape of the pancreas

The shape of the pancreas is variable. Typically it resembles a dumbbell. Sausage and tadpole shapes are also seen (Fig. 7.**13**).

Fig. 7.13 Variants in the shape of the pancreas

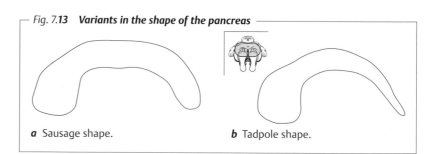

a Sausage shape.

b Tadpole shape.

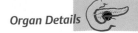

Organ Details

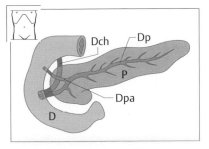

Fig. 7.**14** **Gross anatomy of the pancreas.** D = duodenum, P = pancreas, Dch = common bile duct, Dp = pancreatic duct, Dpa = accessory pancreatic duct.

LEARNING GOALS

➤ Evaluate the echo pattern of the pancreas.
➤ Identify the pancreatic duct.
➤ Identify the common bile duct.
➤ Determine the size of the pancreas.

The pancreas is very rich in parenchyma (pancreas = "all flesh") and has few definable internal structures. The pancreatic duct runs longitudinally through the parenchyma from tail to head, turning downward and backward at the head before joining the common bile duct and opening into the duodenum (Fig. 7.**14**). Ultrasound cannot define the side branches of the duct or an accessory pancreatic duct, if present.

Pancreatic parenchyma

KEY POINT

The parenchyma of the pancreas in young, slender individuals has about the same echogenicity as the liver parenchyma.

The parenchyma in young, slender individuals has a uniform, granular echo texture with approximately the same reflectivity as the liver (Fig. 7.**15**). Its echogenicity is variable, however. It is lower in slender individuals and often increases markedly with ageing and with weight gain (Figs. 7.**16**, 7.**17**). The pancreas then appears as a bright streak lying superficial to the dark splenic vein.

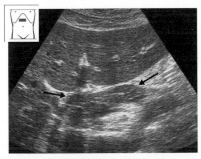

Fig. 7.**15** **Normal pancreas (→←).** Normal pancreatic tissue has about the same echogenicity as the liver.

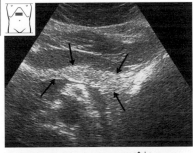

Fig. 7.**16** **Normal pancreas (↑↓) in an elderly subject.** The tissue is relatively echogenic.

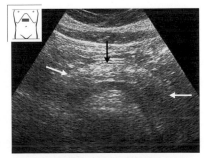

Fig. 7.**17** **Elderly obese subject.** The pancreas (→↓←) is normal and relatively echogenic.

Abnormalities of the pancreatic parenchyma

Fibrolipomatosis. The most common abnormal finding is a homogeneous increase in parenchymal echogenicity due to fatty infiltration in obesity (Figs. 7.**18**, 7.**19**). This condition requires differentiation from a coarse "salt-and-pepper" pattern, which is a normal variant (Fig. 7.**20**).

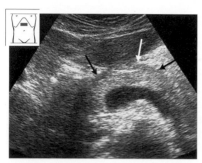

Fig. 7.18 Pancreatic lipomatosis (↓↓↓) in a healthy subject.

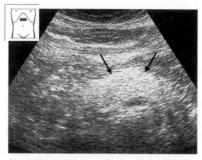

Fig. 7.19 Pancreatic lipomatosis due to alcohol abuse (↓↓). This patient had no known pancreatic disease.

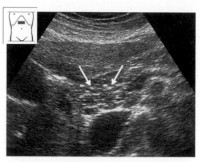

Fig. 7.20 Healthy pancreas, showing a coarse salt-and-pepper echo pattern (↓↓).

Table 7.**1** Sonographic features of chronic pancreatitis

Enlargement of the pancreas

Internal structure coarse and heterogeneous

Calcifications

Pseudocysts

Pancreatic duct dilated

Indistinct contours

Chronic pancreatitis. Chronic pancreatitis is characterized by a coarse, heterogeneous echo pattern of increased density. The changes may be relatively minor (Fig. 7.**21**) or may present as coarse calcifications (Figs. 7.**22**, 7.**23**). The ultrasound features of chronic pancreatitis are listed in Table 7.**1**.

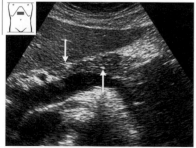

Fig. 7.21 Chronic pancreatitis. Stippled calcifications (↓↑).

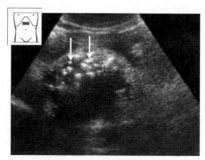

Fig. 7.22 Prominent calcifications, some very coarse (↓↓), in chronic pancreatitis.

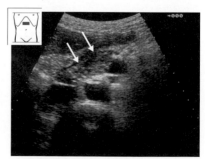

Fig. 7.23 Chronic pancreatitis. Conspicuous calcifications (↓↓).

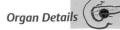

Table 7.**2** Sonographic features of acute pancreatitis

Enlargement of the pancreas
– diffuse
– circumscribed
Internal structure heterogeneous, rarefied, hypoechoic
Indistinct contours

Table 7.**3** Associated findings in acute pancreatitis

Ileus
Ascites
Necrotic tracks
Abscess formation
Bile duct dilatation
Pleural effusion

Acute pancreatitis. Acute pancreatitis leads to homogeneous, hypoechoic swelling of the organ (Figs. 7.24, 7.25). The swelling may be circumscribed or may involve the entire pancreas. There may also be areas of intrapancreatic hemorrhage and necrosis leading to circumscribed, echo-free lesions. Table 7.**2** reviews the sonographic features of acute pancreatitis. Table 7.**3** shows findings that may be seen in association with acute pancreatitis.

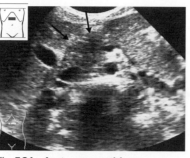

Fig. 7.24 Acute pancreatitis.
Swelling and irregular contours (↓↓).

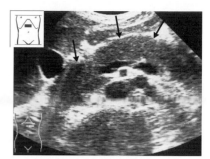

Fig. 7.25 Acute pancreatitis (↓↓↓).

Pseudocysts. Pseudocysts may develop as a complication of acute pancreatitis several weeks after the onset of the disease. Usually these lesions are easy to identify with ultrasound (Figs. 7.**26** – 7.**28**).

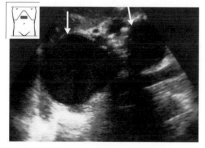

Fig. 7.26 Large pseudocysts (↓↓)
secondary to acute pancreatitis.

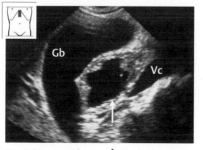

Fig. 7.27 Pseudocyst (↑) in the head of the pancreas. The patient had a history of acute pancreatitis. Gb = gallbladder, Vc = vena cava.

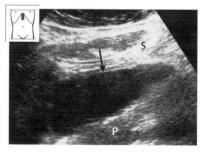

Fig. 7.28 Very large pseudocyst (↓)
following acute pancreatitis.
S = stomach, P = pancreas.

Pancreatic carcinoma. Pancreatic carcinoma most commonly arises in the head of the pancreas. It appears sonographically as a nonhomogeneous, hypoechoic mass. Dilatation of the pancreatic duct is another common finding (see p. 145 and Fig. 7.**29**). It can be very difficult to appreciate a large pancreatic carcinoma due to poor delineation of the pancreas, destruction of the normal architecture, and intervening gas (Figs. 7.**30** – 7.**32**). Table 7.**4** lists the sonographic features of pancreatic carcinoma.

Table 7.**4** Sonographic features of pancreatic carcinoma

Irregular contours

Hypoechoic mass

Dilated pancreatic duct

Infiltration or displacement of surroundings

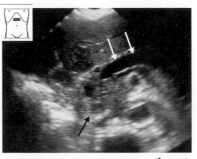

*Fig. 7.29 **Pancreatic carcinoma (↑) with dilatation of the pancreatic duct (↓↓).***

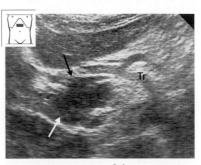

*Fig. 7.30 **Carcinoma of the pancreatic head (↓↑).*** Tr = celiac trunk.

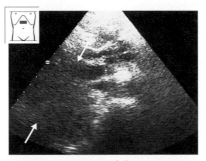

*Fig. 7.31 **Carcinoma of the pancreatic head (↓↑).*** The tumor is 8 cm in diameter. Ultrasound shows only a large, nonhomogeneous, ill-defined mass in the pancreatic region.

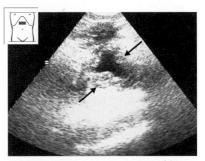

*Fig. 7.32 **Pancreatic carcinoma (↑↓).*** As in Fig. 7.**31**, there is only a vague impression of a partially liquid mass in the pancreatic region.

Pancreatic duct

The pancreatic duct is difficult to define with ultrasound. Start by examining a young, slender subject and optimize the scanning conditions as described above, or you will be disappointed.

It is easiest to define the pancreatic duct in an upper abdominal transverse scan through the body of the pancreas (Fig. 7.**33a**). Locate the duct by scanning across the longitudinal axis of the organ. You may have to do this several times with the transducer placed at slightly different points. Keep in mind that the axis of the pancreas is slightly oblique relative to the transverse axis of the upper abdomen. The duct appears in longitudinal section as a pair of fine, relatively bright wall echoes extending a variable distance through the gland. Figure 7.**33b** shows the appearance of the duct in cross section.

KEY POINTS

The pancreatic duct can be identified as a pair of fine wall echoes.

Its normal diameter is 2–3 mm.

Fig. 7.**33** **Defining the pancreatic duct**

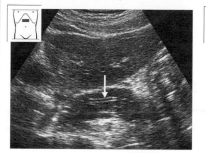

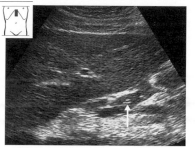

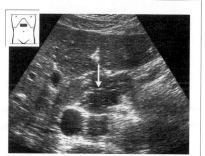

a Longitudinal section of the pancreatic duct (↓) in the body of the pancreas.

b Cross section of the pancreatic duct (↑) in a longitudinal scan through the body of the pancreas.

c Pancreatic duct (↓) in the head of the pancreas. Only a short segment of the duct is seen.

The diameter of the pancreatic duct ranges from 2 to 3 mm (Fig. 7.**34**). Try to track the duct toward the tail and head of the pancreas. Usually you can obtain only a limited view in each direction (Fig. 7.**33c**). The beginner may occasionally mistake the hypoechoic stomach wall for a dilated pancreatic duct (Figs. 7.**35**, 7.**36**). Vessels can also be a source of confusion (Fig. 7.**37**).

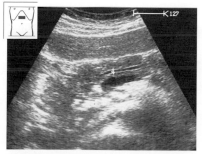

Fig. 7.34 **Measuring the diameter of the pancreatic duct in the body of the pancreas.**

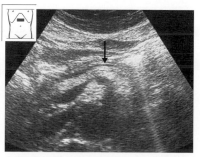

Fig. 7.35 **Hypoechoic stomach wall (↓).** May be confused with the pancreatic duct. Pancreatic lipomatosis.

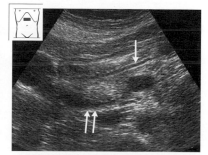

Fig. 7.36 **Hypoechoic stomach wall (↓).** The pancreas (↑↑) is relatively hypoechoic.

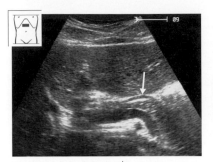

Fig. 7.**37** *Splenic vein (↓) running anterior to the pancreas.*

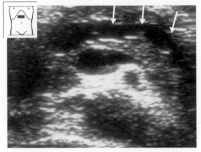

Fig. 7.**38** *Chronic pancreatitis.* A long segment of the pancreatic duct (↓↓↓) can be seen.

Table 7.**5** Differential diagnosis of pancreatic duct dilatation

Chronic pancreatitis

Pancreatic carcinoma

Papillary stenosis

Papillary carcinoma

Bile duct carcinoma

Stones

Abnormalities of the pancreatic duct

In chronic pancreatitis, the pancreatic duct may be somewhat dilated with caliber irregularities (Fig. 7.**38**). Pancreatic carcinoma leads to marked dilatation of the pancreatic duct (see p. 144). Table 7.**5** lists the possible causes of a dilated pancreatic duct.

Common bile duct

You already know the course of the common bile duct through the head of the pancreas (Fig. 7.**14**). Please note that the common bile duct runs down the longitudinal body axis for a considerable distance, lying in the same sagittal plane as the inferior vena cava, which is easily identified with ultrasound. Just before reaching the duodenum, the common duct turns right and a little forward to enter the papilla in the duodenal wall.

Defining the common bile duct in transverse sections

Figure 7.**39** demonstrates the sonographic anatomy of the common bile duct in transverse section.

First define the head of the pancreas in a transverse scan. Acquire a plane that simultaneously displays sections of the gallbladder, duodenum, pancreatic head, and inferior vena cava. This plane will always include a cross section of the common bile duct (Fig. 7.**40 a**). Try to identify the common duct, but do not be discouraged if you are unable to. If you can locate the common duct, picture it as extending out of the image plane. Look again at Fig. 7.**39**. The common bile duct extends toward you from the image plane and enters the second part of the duodenum, which is located just in front of the scan plane. Now move the transducer cephalad in small increments and trace the common duct back toward its origin. You will see the section of the pancreas disappear from the image as you trace the duct up toward the liver (Fig. 7.**40 b**, **c**).

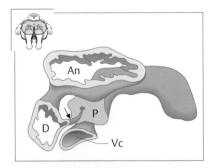

Fig. 7.**39** *Course of the common bile duct in the head of the pancreas.* A transverse scan through the head of the pancreas (P), the second part of the duodenum (D), the antrum (An) and vena cava (Vc) also cuts the common bile duct (↓) transversely in the head of the pancreas. This diagram also shows the duct extending out of the image plane. It turns to the right and enters the second part of the duodenum.

Fig. 7.40 Defining the common bile duct in transverse sections

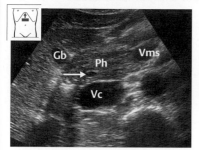 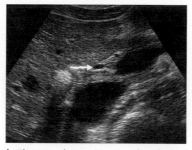 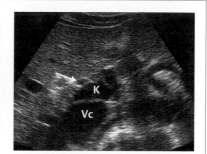

a Transverse scan of the pancreatic head (Ph) between the gallbladder (Gb), vena cava (Vc), and superior mesenteric vein (Vms). The common bile duct (→) is visible in cross section.

b The transducer was moved cephalad, leaving the pancreas behind and showing a higher cross section of the common bile duct (→).

c Scan at a higher level now shows a section of the confluence (K) between the common bile duct (→) and vena cava (Vc). Compare this view with Fig. 7.42 c.

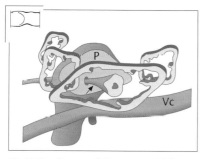

Fig. 7.41 **Course of the common bile duct in longitudinal section.** The scan passes through the head of the pancreas (P), which lies just anterior to the vena cava (Vc). The common bile duct (↑) runs toward you from the image plane. The drawing also shows sections of the duodenal loop and the site where the common duct enters the duodenum.

Defining the common bile duct in longitudinal section

Figure 7.41 demonstrates the sonographic anatomy of the common bile duct in longitudinal section.

Image the head of the pancreas in a transverse scan as before, and identify the section of the common bile duct (Fig. 7.42 a). Now rotate the transducer to a longitudinal scan to obtain an extended longitudinal view of the common duct (Fig. 7.42 b, c).

Fig. 7.42 Defining the common bile duct in longitudinal section

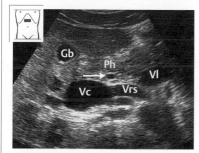 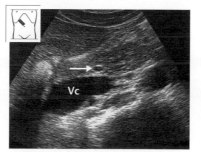 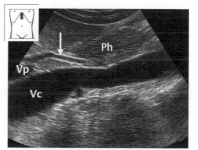

a Transverse scan of the pancreatic head (Ph). Common bile duct (→). Vc = vena cava, Vl = splenic vein, Vrs = left renal vein, Gb = gallbladder.

b The transducer was rotated to a position intermediate between a transverse and longitudinal scan. Common bile duct (→), Vc = vena cava.

c The transducer is placed sagittally over the vena cava (Vc). You see the pancreatic head (Ph) and common bile duct (↓) plus a section of the portal vein (Vp). Compare this view with Fig. 7.40 c.

Abnormalities of the common bile duct within the pancreas

An obstruction of the common bile duct can cause significant dilatation that includes the intrapancreatic segment of the duct (Fig. 7.**43**).

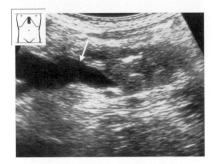

Fig. 7.**43** **Carcinoma of the pancreatic head.** The common bile duct is obstructed and greatly dilated (↓). Compare with Fig. 7.**42 c**.

Measuring the pancreatic diameter

KEY POINT

The diameter of the pancreas ranges from 2.5 cm in the body to 3.5 cm at the head.

The different parts of the pancreas vary considerably in size. The diameters of the head, body, and tail are determined by measuring the maximum cross-sectional dimension perpendicular to the long axis of the organ (Fig. 7.**44**). The following dimensions are considered normal:

➤ Head 3.5 cm
➤ Body 2.5 cm
➤ Tail 3.0 cm

Fig. 7.**44** **Measuring the diameter of the pancreas**

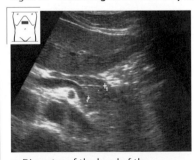

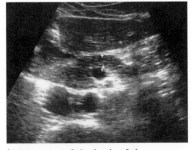

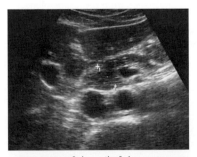

a Diameter of the head of the pancreas.

b Diameter of the body of the pancreas.

c Diameter of the tail of the pancreas.

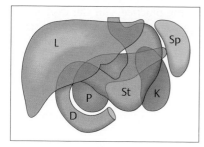

 # Anatomical Relationships

With a length of approximately 15 cm and a diameter of 2–3 cm, the pancreas is related to numerous organs in its course through the upper abdomen (Fig. 7.**45**). We will therefore consider its relationships separately for the tail, body, and head.

Relationships of the tail of the pancreas

Fig. 7.45 Relationships of the pancreas. L = liver, D = duodenum, P = pancreas, K = kidney, Sp = spleen, St = stomach.

The tail of the pancreas is related to the following organs (Fig. 7.**46**):
➤ Anteriorly: body of the stomach and left lobe of the liver
➤ Posteriorly: left kidney and splenic vein
➤ Superiorly: body and cardia of the stomach
➤ Inferiorly: jejunum
➤ Laterally: colon and splenic hilum

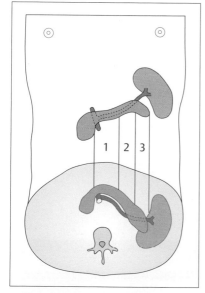

Fig. 7.47 Course of the splenic vein in relation to the body and tail of the pancreas. The body of the pancreas lies anterior to the splenic vein (segment 1). The pancreas and splenic vein then run posteriorly to the left of the spinal column (segment 2). The pancreas is still anterior and the splenic vein posterior. After that the splenic vein continues to run laterally but not posteriorly, while the pancreas extends farther posteriorly and a little inferiorly (segment 3).

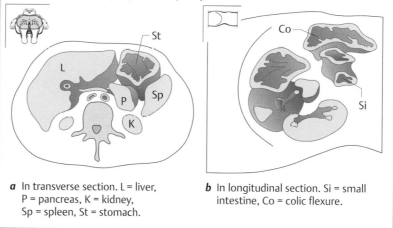

Fig. 7.46 Relationships of the tail of the pancreas

a In transverse section. L = liver, P = pancreas, K = kidney, Sp = spleen, St = stomach.

b In longitudinal section. Si = small intestine, Co = colic flexure.

Note that while the splenic vein runs behind the body of the pancreas, it lies superior to the pancreatic tail. This relationship can be difficult to understand; it is illustrated in Fig. 7.**47**.

Relationship of the pancreatic tail to the spleen, and the transsplenic approach to scanning the tail

As you have seen, the tail of the pancreas extends quite far posteriorly. Therefore it cannot be adequately scanned from the front of the abdomen in either transverse or longitudinal planes. With some practice, you can exploit the proximity of the spleen and utilize that organ as an acoustic window for scanning the tail of the pancreas (Fig. 7.**48**).

Transverse scanning of the pancreatic tail through the spleen

Position the transducer for a transverse flank scan, approximately on the posterior axillary line, and demonstrate the spleen (Fig. 7.**48 b**). Then move the scan plane slightly lower. A section of the upper pole of the kidney will appear on the right side of the screen. Also identify the splenic vein at the hilum of the spleen (Fig. 7.**48 c**). You know that the tail of the pancreas lies just caudal to the splenic vein at this level. Now move the transducer slightly lower, and you can identify the tail of the pancreas in the triangle between the spleen and kidney (Fig. 7.**48 d**).

Fig. 7.48 *Transverse scanning of the pancreatic tail through the spleen*

a Transverse scan from the left flank passes through the kidney (K), spleen (Sp), and pancreatic tail (Pt). The rest of the pancreas is shown in front of the image plane to clarify the scan location. Splenic vein (←).

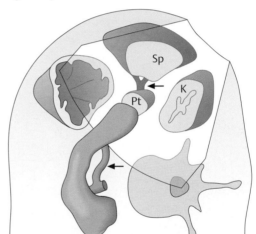

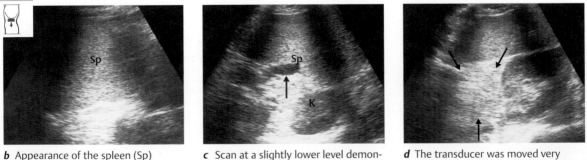

b Appearance of the spleen (Sp) in the transverse flank scan.

c Scan at a slightly lower level demonstrates the superior pole of the kidney (K), the spleen (Sp), and the splenic vein (↑).

d The transducer was moved very slightly caudad. The tail of the pancreas (↓↓↑) can now be identified between the spleen and kidney.

Longitudinal scanning of the pancreatic tail through the spleen

The coronal section in Fig. 7.**49 a** shows how the spleen and the tail of the pancreas are displayed in the longitudinal flank scan. First image the kidney and spleen in a longitudinal scan from the flank (Fig. 7.**49 b**). Note the position of the transducer. Angle the scan slightly upward, then slowly move the transducer anteriorly until you see the upper pole of the kidney and a section of the spleen (Fig. 7.**49 c**). When you now angle the probe a little farther anteriorly, the kidney will disappear from the image. In its place you will see the tail of the pancreas, which lies medial to the spleen and caudal to the splenic vein (Fig. 7.**49 d**).

Fig. 7.49   Longitudinal scanning of the pancreatic tail through the spleen

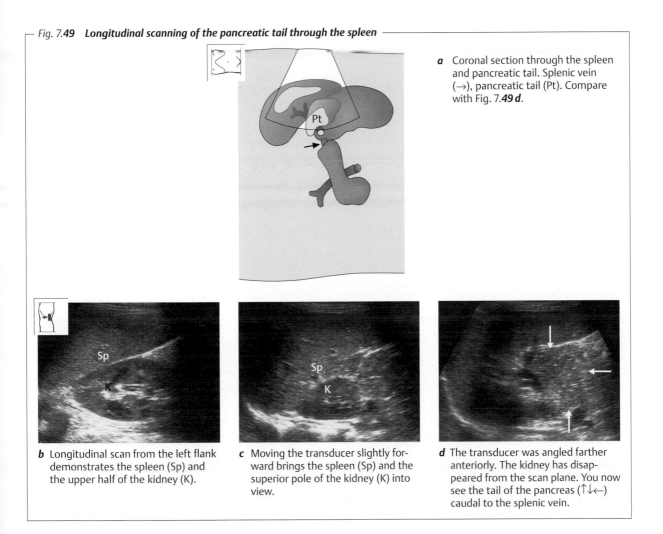

a Coronal section through the spleen and pancreatic tail. Splenic vein (→), pancreatic tail (Pt). Compare with Fig. 7.**49 d**.

b Longitudinal scan from the left flank demonstrates the spleen (Sp) and the upper half of the kidney (K).

c Moving the transducer slightly forward brings the spleen (Sp) and the superior pole of the kidney (K) into view.

d The transducer was angled farther anteriorly. The kidney has disappeared from the scan plane. You now see the tail of the pancreas (↑↓←) caudal to the splenic vein.

Relationships of the body of the pancreas _____

The body of the pancreas is related to the following organs (Fig. 7.**50**):
➤ Anteriorly: left lobe of the liver and antrum of the stomach
➤ Posteriorly: splenic vein, confluence, superior mesenteric artery, and splenic artery
➤ Superiorly: celiac trunk
➤ Inferiorly: jejunum

You have already seen how the retroperitoneal vessels are used as landmarks for locating the pancreas.

Fig. 7. ***50*** **Relationships of the head of the pancreas**

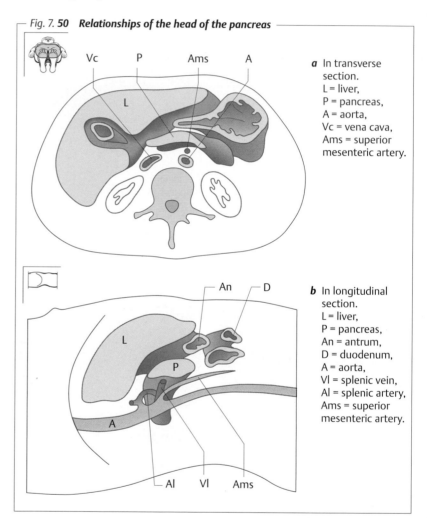

a In transverse section.
L = liver,
P = pancreas,
A = aorta,
Vc = vena cava,
Ams = superior mesenteric artery.

b In longitudinal section.
L = liver,
P = pancreas,
An = antrum,
D = duodenum,
A = aorta,
Vl = splenic vein,
Al = splenic artery,
Ams = superior mesenteric artery.

Relationship of the body of the pancreas to the stomach and liver

The stomach creates most of the problems encountered in scanning the pancreas (Fig. 7.**51**). The worst-case situation is when the stomach contains a mixture of solid material, liquid, and gas. It is best to examine subjects early in the morning or after they have swallowed 0.5 to 1 liter of water.

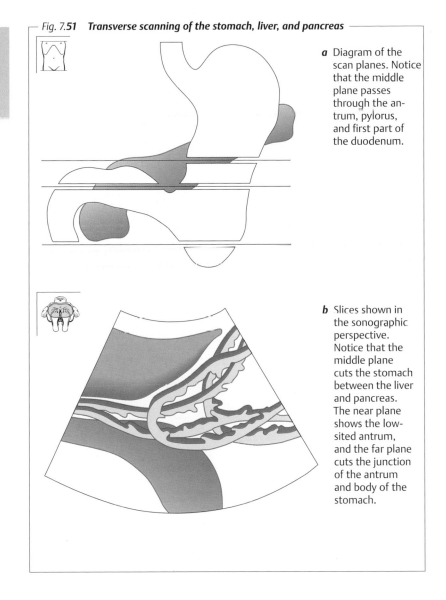

Fig. 7.51 **Transverse scanning of the stomach, liver, and pancreas**

a Diagram of the scan planes. Notice that the middle plane passes through the antrum, pylorus, and first part of the duodenum.

b Slices shown in the sonographic perspective. Notice that the middle plane cuts the stomach between the liver and pancreas. The near plane shows the low-sited antrum, and the far plane cuts the junction of the antrum and body of the stomach.

Defining the relations of the pancreatic body to the stomach and liver in transverse sections

Place the probe transversely over the pancreas and identify the pancreas, splenic vein, superior mesenteric artery, and aorta. Picture where you would expect to find the stomach: at the right edge of the image, in the junctional area between the body and tail of the pancreas. This low portion of the stomach consists of the antrum (Fig. 7.**52 a**) and its junction with the body of the stomach. Most of the body of the stomach lies against the anterior surface of the pancreas. Now slide the transducer a little lower. Notice how the stomach passes between the pancreas and liver (Fig. 7.**52 b**). This portion consists of the antrum, the prepyloric antrum, and its junction with the duodenal bulb. As you move the transducer lower from there, the pancreas disappears from the image and the low part of the antrum comes into view (Fig. 7.**52 c**).

Fig. 7.52   Defining the relationships of the pancreatic body to the stomach and liver in transverse sections
(The scan planes correspond to those in Fig. 7.**51**.)

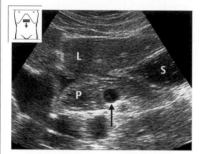

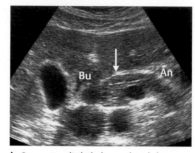

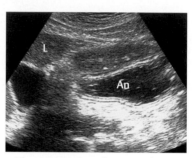

a Scan at the level of the pancreatic body. P = pancreas, St = stomach, L = liver, confluence (↑).

b Scan at a slightly lower level demonstrates the antrum (An) and duodenal bulb (Bu) with the apposed stomach walls (↓) between them.

c The pancreas is no longer in the scan plane. You see only sections of the antrum (An) and liver (L).

Defining the relation of the pancreatic body to the stomach and liver in longitudinal sections

Demonstrate the liver and the fluid-filled stomach in an upper abdominal longitudinal scan. Identify the pancreas behind the liver. Scan across the liver, stomach, and body of the pancreas in parallel longitudinal sections (Figs. 7.**53**, 7.**54**).

Fig. 7.53   *Longitudinal survey of the stomach, liver, and pancreas*

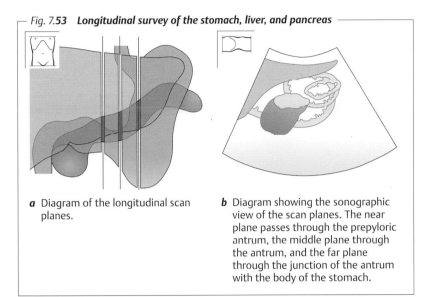

a Diagram of the longitudinal scan planes.

b Diagram showing the sonographic view of the scan planes. The near plane passes through the prepyloric antrum, the middle plane through the antrum, and the far plane through the junction of the antrum with the body of the stomach.

Fig. 7.54   *Defining the relationships of the pancreatic body to the stomach and liver in longitudinal sections*

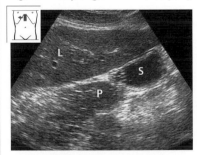
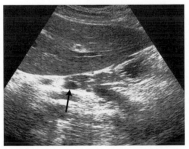
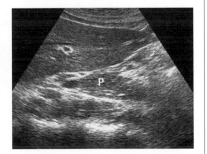

a Scan through the stomach (St), liver (L), and pancreas (P).

b The transducer was moved slightly to the right. A more extended section of the pancreatic head is seen. Splenic vein (↑).

c Section in the region of the pylorus. A gastric lumen is no longer clearly identified. P = pancreas.

Relationships of the head of the pancreas

Figure 7.**55** shows the topographic anatomy of the pancreatic head, which you already know. The relations of the pancreatic head are as follows:
➤ Anteriorly: pyloric region, duodenal bulb, and liver
➤ Posteriorly: vena cava and right renal vein
➤ Superiorly: portal vein and hepatic artery
➤ Inferiorly: third part of the duodenum
➤ Laterally: second part of the duodenum
➤ Medially: superior mesenteric vein
➤ The pancreatic head is also traversed by the common bile duct.

The topographic relationships of the pancreatic head are more complex than those of the body and tail. Figure 7.**56** demonstrates this in transverse and longitudinal sections.

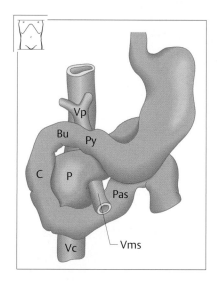

Fig. 7.**55** **Topographic anatomy of the pancreatic head.** P = pancreas, Py = pylorus, Bu = duodenal bulb, C = second part of the duodenum, Pas = third part of the duodenum, Vc = vena cava, Vp = portal vein, Vms = superior mesenteric vein.

Fig. 7.**56** **Relationships of the pancreatic head**

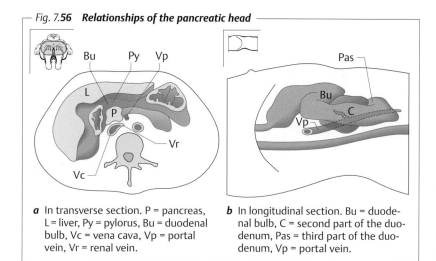

a In transverse section. P = pancreas, L = liver, Py = pylorus, Bu = duodenal bulb, Vc = vena cava, Vp = portal vein, Vr = renal vein.

b In longitudinal section. Bu = duodenal bulb, C = second part of the duodenum, Pas = third part of the duodenum, Vp = portal vein.

Relationships of the pancreatic head to the vena cava, portal vein, splenic vein, and superior mesenteric vein

The vena cava runs parallel to the longitudinal body axis. It is related posteriorly to the pancreatic head. Thus, the spatial relationship of the pancreatic head to the vena cava is relatively easy to understand and demonstrate with ultrasound. Its relationships to the portal vein, splenic vein, and superior mesenteric vein are somewhat more complicated. In the frontal view, the portal vein runs at about a 45° angle to the longitudinal body axis. The superior mesenteric vein runs at a slight angle, and the splenic vein runs a tortuous course at almost a 90° angle to the superior mesenteric vein (Fig. 7.**57**).

Fig. 7.57 *Relationship of the pancreatic head to the vena cava, portal vein, splenic vein, and superior mesenteric vein*

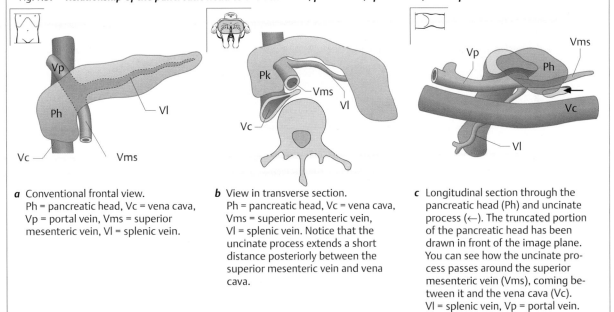

a Conventional frontal view.
Ph = pancreatic head, Vc = vena cava, Vp = portal vein, Vms = superior mesenteric vein, Vl = splenic vein.

b View in transverse section.
Ph = pancreatic head, Vc = vena cava, Vms = superior mesenteric vein, Vl = splenic vein. Notice that the uncinate process extends a short distance posteriorly between the superior mesenteric vein and vena cava.

c Longitudinal section through the pancreatic head (Ph) and uncinate process (←). The truncated portion of the pancreatic head has been drawn in front of the image plane. You can see how the uncinate process passes around the superior mesenteric vein (Vms), coming between it and the vena cava (Vc). Vl = splenic vein, Vp = portal vein.

Defining the relationships of the pancreatic head to the vena cava, portal vein, splenic vein, and superior mesenteric vein in transverse sections

Position the transducer for an upper abdominal transverse scan and identify the pancreas with its landmark, the superior mesenteric vein. Move the transducer caudad in small, parallel steps and watch the sections of the pancreas and splenic vein. The longitudinal section of the splenic vein (Fig. 7.**58a**) widens to become the confluence (Fig. 7.**58 b**), which in turn merges with the superior mesenteric vein (Fig. 7.**58 c**). Unlike the splenic vein, the superior mesenteric vein presents a rounded cross section in the transverse scan. Meanwhile, the slender body of the pancreas is replaced by the broader head.

Fig. 7.58   *Relationship of the pancreatic head to the splenic vein, confluence, and superior mesenteric vein in transverse sections*

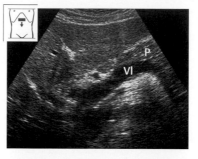

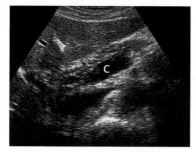

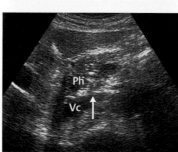

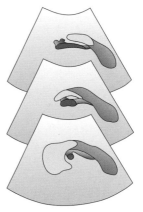

a   Transverse scan at a relatively high level displays a longitudinal section of the pancreatic head (P) and splenic vein (Vl).

b The scan was moved slightly lower. The splenic vein gives way to the thicker confluence (C) of the superior mesenteric and splenic veins.

c Scan at a lower level displays the pancreatic head (Ph) and uncinate process. The superior mesenteric vein (↑) is visible in cross section. Note that the uncinate process passes around the superior mesenteric vein. Vc = vena cava.

d Diagram of the scan planes in *a–c*.

Defining the relationships of the pancreatic head to the vena cava, portal vein, superior mesenteric vein, and splenic vein in longitudinal sections

Position the transducer for an upper abdominal transverse scan and define the pancreatic head with its landmark, the splenic vein. Rotate the transducer under vision to a longitudinal scan, and identify the cross section of the splenic vein and, anterior to it, the section of the pancreas. Slide the transducer to the right in small increments. Observe the sections of the pancreas and splenic vein. First you will see the round cross section of the splenic vein posterior to the pancreas (Fig. 7.**59 a**). As you move the transducer to the right, you will see the splenic vein give way to the confluence, which merges with a longitudinal section of the superior mesenteric vein (Fig. 7.**59 b**). Scanning farther to the right, you will see the confluence give way to the portal vein, whose section is now cranial to the broad head of the pancreas (Fig. 7.**59 c**).

Fig. 7.59   Relationship of pancreatic head to splenic vein, confluence, and superior mesenteric vein in longitudinal sections

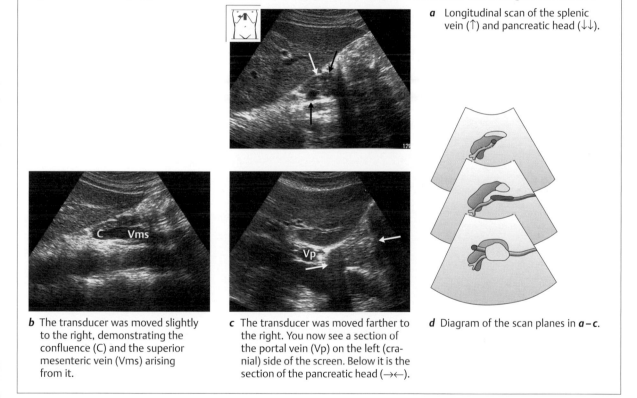

a Longitudinal scan of the splenic vein (↑) and pancreatic head (↓↓).

b The transducer was moved slightly to the right, demonstrating the confluence (C) and the superior mesenteric vein (Vms) arising from it.

c The transducer was moved farther to the right. You now see a section of the portal vein (Vp) on the left (cranial) side of the screen. Below it is the section of the pancreatic head (→←).

d Diagram of the scan planes in **a–c**.

Relationship of the pancreatic head to the duodenum

You know how the pancreatic head is related to the duodenal loop in the classic frontal view (Fig. 7.55). Notice that the pyloric region lies anterior to the junction of the pancreatic head and body. The second part of the duodenum is lateral to the pancreatic head, which fits within the loop of the duodenum. Figure 7.**60** shows the sonographic perspective in transverse and longitudinal sections.

Fig. 7.**60**   *Topography of the pancreatic head*

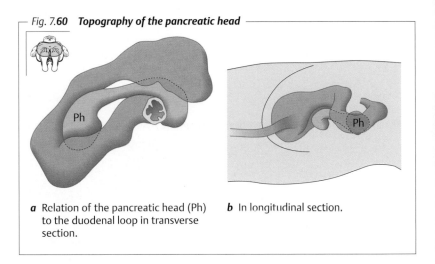

a Relation of the pancreatic head (Ph) to the duodenal loop in transverse section.

b In longitudinal section.

Defining the relation of the pancreatic head to the duodenum in transverse sections

Define the pancreatic head in an upper abdominal transverse scan. It is located just anterior to the vena cava. Slowly move the transducer caudad. You will see the pancreas disappear, being replaced by an irregular echo pattern. Recognize what causes this: it is the third part of the duodenum, which lies below the pancreatic head. Now return to the original plane. What do you expect to find to the right of the pancreatic head? The second part of the duodenum, i.e., a cross section through the middle of the duodenal loop. Now move the scan higher and consider what you would expect to find anterior to the pancreatic head: the duodenal bulb and antrum. Make several cranial-to-caudal passes from this level while watching the sections of the duodenal bulb and the second and third parts of the duodenum. The typical appearances are shown in Figs. 7.61 and 7.62.

Fig. 7.61 *Relationship of the pancreatic head to the duodenum in transverse sections*

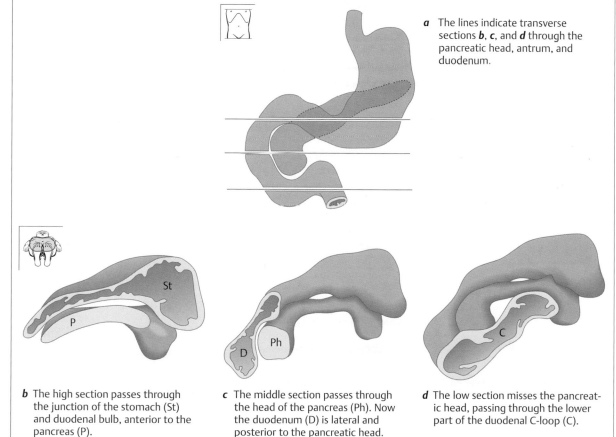

a The lines indicate transverse sections *b*, *c*, and *d* through the pancreatic head, antrum, and duodenum.

b The high section passes through the junction of the stomach (St) and duodenal bulb, anterior to the pancreas (P).

c The middle section passes through the head of the pancreas (Ph). Now the duodenum (D) is lateral and posterior to the pancreatic head.

d The low section misses the pancreatic head, passing through the lower part of the duodenal C-loop (C).

Fig. 7.62 Defining the relationship of the pancreatic head to the antrum and duodenum in transverse sections

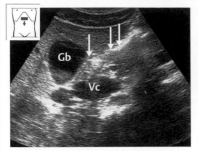

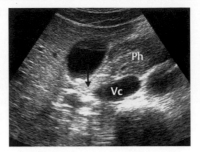

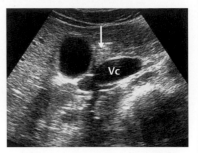

a The high section passes through the duodenum (↓) and the junction of the stomach (↓↓) and duodenal bulb. Gb = gallbladder, Vc = vena cava.

b Section of the pancreatic head (Pk), which directly overlies the vena cava (Vc). A section of the second part of the duodenum (↓) appears between the vena cava and gallbladder.

c The low section passes through the vena cava (Vc) and the overlying third part of the duodenum (↓).

Defining the relationship of the pancreatic head to the duodenum in longitudinal sections

Define the pancreatic head in a longitudinal scan. Identify the triad of the liver, pancreas, and duodenal bulb (Figs. 7.**63 b**, 7.**64 a**). Scan slowly to the right in parallel sections. As you do so, watch the sections of the duodenum and pancreas. At first the duodenal bulb lies anterior to the pancreas. As you slide the transducer to the right, the section of the duodenum moves cephalad and posteriorly (Figs. 7.**63 c**, 7.**64 b**). As you continue scanning to the right, the pancreas disappears from the image rather abruptly, and in its place you see the irregular pattern of the air- and fluid-filled second part of the duodenum (Figs. 7.**63 d**, 7.**64 c**).

Generally this sequence of images is difficult to acquire. It can be helpful to fill the stomach with 1 liter of water and follow the liquid as it is periodically emptied into the duodenum. It may also help to examine the subject in a standing position. Keep in mind that the duodenal lumen can present to the examiner in three ways:
➤ hypoechoic = fluid-filled,
➤ white = air-filled,
➤ nonhomogeneous = mixed.

Of course, these phenomena may be seen concurrently at adjacent sites in the duodenum and may show peristaltic changes. As a result, examination of the pancreatic head and its surroundings can be a very difficult and time-consuming process for the beginner.

Fig. 7.63 *Relationship of the pancreatic head to the duodenum in longitudinal sections*

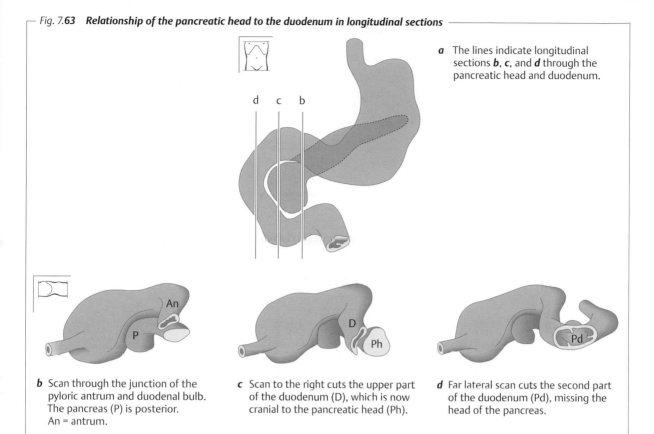

a The lines indicate longitudinal sections **b**, **c**, and **d** through the pancreatic head and duodenum.

b Scan through the junction of the pyloric antrum and duodenal bulb. The pancreas (P) is posterior. An = antrum.

c Scan to the right cuts the upper part of the duodenum (D), which is now cranial to the pancreatic head (Ph).

d Far lateral scan cuts the second part of the duodenum (Pd), missing the head of the pancreas.

Fig. 7.64 *Defining the relationship of the pancreatic head to the duodenum in longitudinal sections*

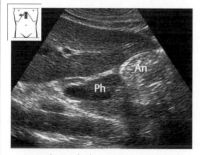
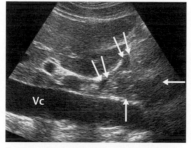
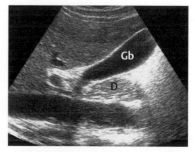

a Scan through the antrum (An) and pancreatic head (Ph).

b The transducer was moved slightly to the right. The duodenum runs cephalad and posteriorly (↓↓). The pancreatic head (↑←) directly overlies the vena cava (Vc).

c Scan farther to the right misses the pancreatic head but cuts the second part of the duodenum (D) and also the gallbladder (Gb).

8 Stomach, Duodenum, and Diaphragm

LEARNING GOALS

➤ Identify the stomach and duodenum.
➤ Identify the area of the diaphragm pierced by the aorta and vena cava.

TIP

The liver provides an acoustic window for scanning the stomach and duodenum.

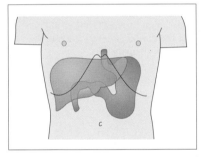

Fig. 8.1 Frontal view of the stomach and duodenum.

The stomach and duodenum are usually considered barriers to scanning and are not always specifically identified and examined as objects of interest. While it is true that the stomach and duodenum are not classic ultrasound organs, often they are not too difficult to examine, even without special patient preparations, if you know where to look. Of course, gastrointestinal scanning is basically a task for the advanced sonographer. However, we include the stomach and bowel in this introduction to emphasize that they are not merely obstacles but are part of the upper abdominal anatomy that is accessible to deliberate examination. At the same time, we would advise beginners to be very cautious in interpreting their findings.

A familiarity with the diaphragm in the area where it is pierced by the aorta and vena cava is of some importance, since the diaphragm in that area may be confused with the right adrenal gland or may be misinterpreted as a vascular structure.

Figure 8.1 shows an anterior view of the stomach and duodenum as they appear in anatomical textbooks.

The structures that often can be seen clearly with ultrasound are the cardia and gastroesophageal junction, the antrum, and the first and second parts of the duodenum (Figs. 8.2, 8.3). The liver provides an acoustic window for scanning these structures. It is far more difficult to obtain a clear view of the fundus and body of the stomach by scanning from the front of the abdomen or through the spleen.

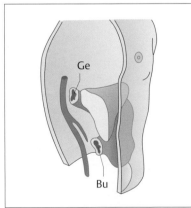

Fig. 8.2 Oblique longitudinal scan. This plane demonstrates the gastroesophageal junction (Ge) and the junction of the stomach and duodenal bulb (Bu).

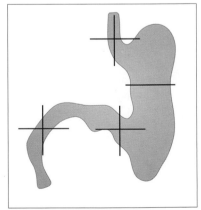

Fig. 8.3 Scan planes for demonstrating the stomach and duodenum.

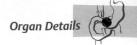

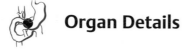 # Organ Details

Stomach wall

If the scanner has good resolution and conditions are favorable, five layers can be distinguished in the stomach wall (Fig. 8.**4**):
➤ The echogenic interface between the lumen and mucosa
➤ The hypoechoic muscularis mucosae
➤ The echogenic submucosa
➤ The hypoechoic muscularis externa
➤ The echogenic outer surface of the serosa

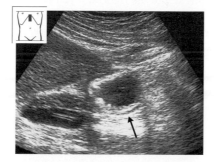

Fig. 8.4 **The layered structure of the stomach wall (↑).**

These five layers cannot always be clearly identified, however. The best section for this purpose is one through the antrum. Often only three layers can be recognized: the echogenic inner and outer layers and the hypoechoic middle layer (as shown in Fig. 8.**21 a**).

Changes in the stomach wall

It would be beyond our scope to explore the ultrasound diagnosis of benign and malignant changes in the stomach wall. Figure 8.**5** shows an example of a stomach wall lesion that can be identified with ultrasound.

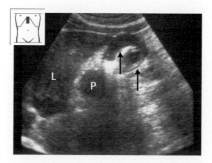

Fig. 8.5 **Gastric carcinoma.** Asymmetrical, hypoechoic expansion of the stomach wall in the antral region (↑). L = liver, P = pancreas.

Organ Boundaries and Relationships

Esophagus and cardia

Defining the gastroesophageal junction in longitudinal section

Generally the cardia is best demonstrated in an upper abdominal longitudinal scan that displays the stomach between the liver and the aorta. Center the transducer very high in the epigastrium (Fig. 8.**6 b**). Visualize the aorta. Now angle the transducer to scan longitudinally into the upper abdomen. Tilt it slightly to the right, and you will obtain an elongated section of the esophagus (Fig. 8.**6 a**). Now angle the transducer to the left, and you will see the esophagus merge with the gastric cardia (Fig. 8.**6 c**).

*Fig. 8.**6*** *Defining the gastroesophageal junction in longitudinal sections*

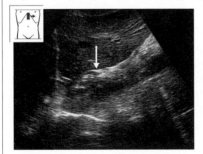
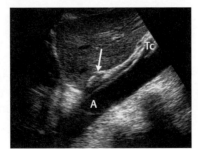
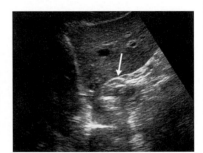

a Elongated section of the abdominal esophagus (↓).

b Scanning a little to the left shows a rounded section of the abdominal esophagus (↓) just above the cardia. A = aorta, Tc = celiac trunk.

c Scan farther to the left. The esophagus has united with the cardia (↓).

Relationships of the esophagus and cardia

Figure 8.**7** illustrates the structures that surround the gastroesophageal junction.

Fig. 8.**7**   *Relations of the esophagus and cardia in transverse and longitudinal sections*

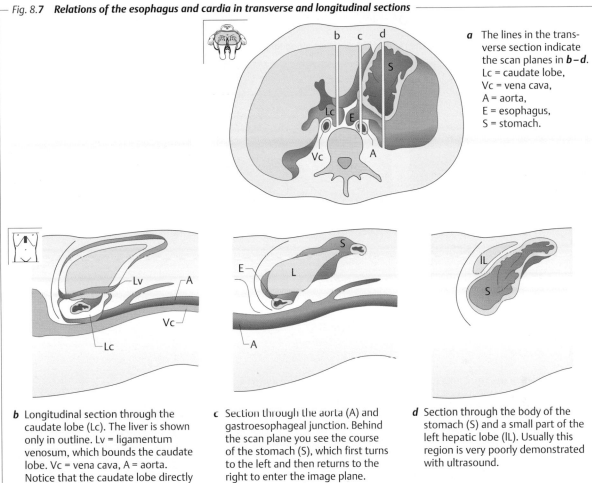

a The lines in the transverse section indicate the scan planes in **b–d**.
Lc = caudate lobe,
Vc = vena cava,
A = aorta,
E = esophagus,
S = stomach.

b Longitudinal section through the caudate lobe (Lc). The liver is shown only in outline. Lv = ligamentum venosum, which bounds the caudate lobe. Vc = vena cava, A = aorta. Notice that the caudate lobe directly overlies the vena cava, coming between that vessel and the esophagus.

c Section through the aorta (A) and gastroesophageal junction. Behind the scan plane you see the course of the stomach (S), which first turns to the left and then returns to the right to enter the image plane. L = liver, E = esophagus.

d Section through the body of the stomach (S) and a small part of the left hepatic lobe (IL). Usually this region is very poorly demonstrated with ultrasound.

Scan longitudinally over the aorta and display the familiar section (Fig. 8.**8 a**). Slide the transducer to the right in small increments. Watch as the section of the aorta disappears and the well-defined caudate lobe of the liver comes into view (Fig. 8.**8 b**). Move the transducer farther to the right, displaying the vena cava in longitudinal section (Fig. 8.**8 c**).

Fig. 8.8   *Defining the structures to the right of the gastroesophageal junction*

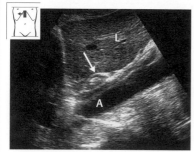
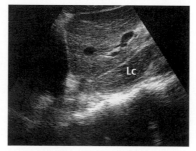
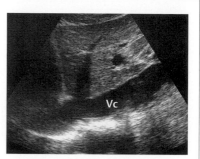

a Scan of the esophagus (↓), liver (L), and aorta (A).

b Scan slightly to the right demonstrates the caudate lobe (Lc).

c Scan farther to the right demonstrates the vena cava (Vc).

Return to the starting point and continue past it toward the left side. See how the esophagus merges with the cardia, and the cardia with the body of the stomach (Fig. 8.**9**).

Fig. 8.9   *Defining the structures to the left of the gastroesophageal junction*

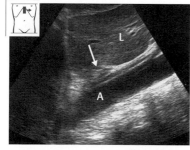
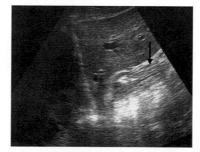
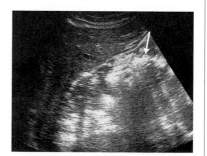

a Scan of the esophagus (↓), liver (L), and aorta (A).

b Scan slightly to the left. The esophagus has merged with the cardia (↓).

c Scan farther to the left demonstrates the body of the stomach (↓) with its heterogeneous contents.

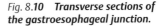

Defining the gastroesophageal junction in transverse sections

Figure 8.**10** shows serial transverse sections of the gastroesophageal junction. With the transducer placed transversely on the upper abdomen, identify the aorta, vena cava, and gastroesophageal junction (Fig. 8.**11 a**). Now move the transducer caudad in parallel transverse scans (Fig. 8.**11 b, c**). Observe the changing shape of the esophagus. Its lumen is round at the site where it pierces the diaphragm. Just below that level it widens toward the left (toward the right on the screen) and opens into the stomach. The cardia presents a horn-shaped cross section. Angle the transducer back and forth several times at this level and trace the opening of the esophagus toward the cardia. Try to gain a three-dimensional impression of this junctional region.

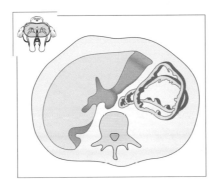

*Fig. 8.**10*** ***Transverse sections of the gastroesophageal junction.***

*Fig. 8.**11*** ***Defining the gastroesophageal junction in transverse sections***

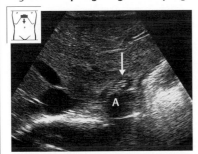

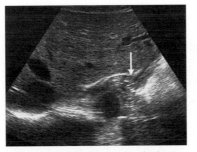

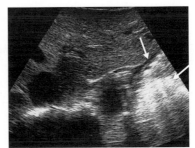

a Transverse scan of the esophagus (↓) just anterior to the aorta (A).

b Scan at a slightly lower level. The cardia (↓) opens to the left.

c Scan below the level in ***b*** displays a nonhomogeneous section of the body of the stomach (↓←).

Body of the stomach

Defining the body of the stomach in longitudinal sections

When the subject has not been specially prepared, the body of the stomach appears only as a heterogeneous region behind the left lobe of the liver. This region is easy to identify by starting from the gastroesophageal junction. We will not go into a detailed evaluation at this introductory level. Figure 8.**12** shows the course of the body of the stomach in longitudinal section.

Scan longitudinally over the left lobe of the liver and the gastroesophageal junction. Move the transducer toward the left side in small increments (Fig. 8.**13**). Observe the expansion of the gastric lumen.

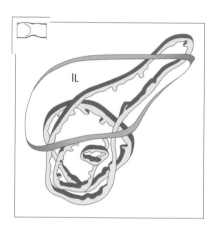

Fig. 8.12   Longitudinal slices of the body of the stomach. You see the section of the left hepatic lobe (IL, shown only in outline) and of the gastroesophageal junction. Behind it (laterally), the gastric lumen expands to form the main body of the stomach.

―― *Fig. 8.13   Defining the body of the stomach in longitudinal sections* ――

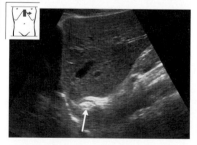

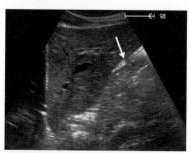

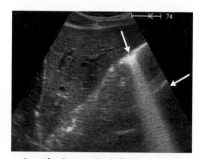

a Longitudinal scan through the liver and gastroesophageal junction (↑).

b The transducer was moved to the left. The stomach (↓) expands.

c Scan farther to the left demonstrates the broad gastric lumen (↓←) with its mixed solid and gaseous contents.

Defining the body of the stomach in transverse sections

Start with a transverse section through the gastroesophageal junction and scan down the body of the stomach. Figures 8.**14** and 8.**15** show the course of the stomach in transverse section.

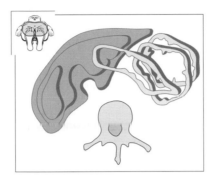

*Fig. 8.**14*** *** Transverse sections through the body of the stomach.***

---

*Fig. 8.**15*** ** *Defining the body of the stomach in transverse sections***

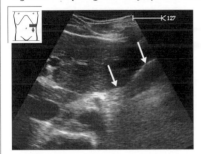 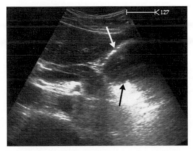 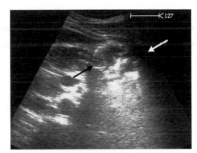

a Relatively high transverse scan through the body of the stomach (↓↓).

b The transducer was moved to a lower level. Body of the stomach (↑↓).

c The transducer was moved lower. Body of the stomach (→←).

Filling the body of the stomach with fluid

Identification of the stomach is made much easier by filling the organ with fluid.

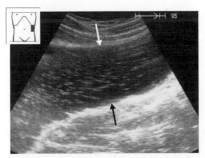 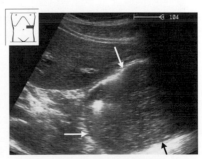

*Fig. 8.**16*** * Longitudinal scan through the fluid-filled body of the stomach (↑↓).*

*Fig. 8.**17*** * Transverse scan through the fluid-filled body of the stomach (→↓↑).*

Antrum and duodenum

Defining the antrum and duodenum in longitudinal sections

Like the cardia, the gastric antrum can be clearly identified with ultrasound in many patients. The shape and size of the stomach are highly variable, but the antrum is found fairly consistently just to the left of the midline behind the liver (Fig. 8.**18**).

Place the transducer longitudinally just to the left of the midline, directly below the costal margin. Display the inferior border of the liver so that it just reaches the right half of the screen. Look for the ringlike structure of the antrum. Figure 8.**19 a** shows the typical appearance.

When you have identified the antrum, hold the transducer very still and observe the spontaneous peristaltic motion. Picture what lies behind the image plane: the portion of the antrum that extends laterally and posteriorly.

Move the transducer to the left in parallel longitudinal scans and observe how the image changes (Fig. 8.**19 b, c**). The ringlike structure of the antrum is lost, and the inferior border of the liver disappears from the screen. The well-ordered structures are replaced by the heterogeneous echo pattern of the stomach, containing air, fluid, and food residues.

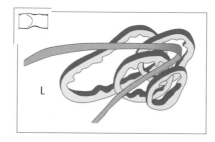

*Fig. 8.**18** Longitudinal slices of the antrum.* The liver (L) is shown only in outline. The near slice passes through the liver and antrum. Additional slices of the antrum are shown behind (lateral to) the near plane.

Fig. 8.**19** *Defining the antrum in longitudinal sections*

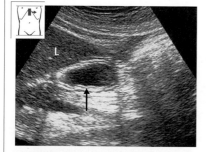

a Longitudinal scan through the antrum (↑) and liver (L).

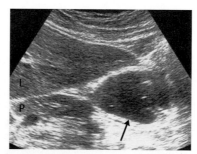

b The transducer was moved slightly to the left. The antrum (↑) expands. L = liver, P = pancreas.

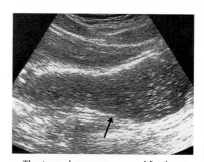

c The transducer was moved farther to the left. The antrum merges with the body of the stomach (↑).

Now return to the starting point over the antrum. Picture what you would expect to find in front of the image plane (Fig. 8.**20**). Just this side of the antrum is the pyloric region, which connects to the duodenal bulb. This first part of the duodenum runs slightly upward, backward, and laterally and finally merges with the second part of the duodenum (Fig. 8.**21**).

Move the transducer to the right in small, parallel steps and observe the course of the duodenum. First it is related to the inferior border of the liver, where it is identified as a very nonhomogeneous structure. As you move farther to the right, a section of the gallbladder comes between the liver and duodenum and then disappears from view, being replaced by a longitudinal section of the second part of the duodenum. The duodenum is very nonhomogeneous and is difficult to distinguish from its surroundings.

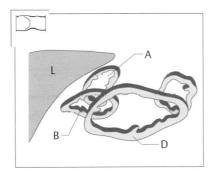

*Fig. 8.**20*** ***Longitudinal slices of the antrum and duodenum.*** The far plane cuts the liver (L) and antrum (A) as shown in Fig. 8.***19a***. The other planes cut the duodenal bulb (B) and the second part of the duodenum (D).

*Fig. 8.**21*** ***Defining the antrum and duodenum in longitudinal sections***

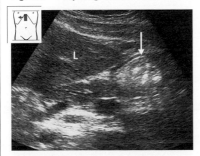

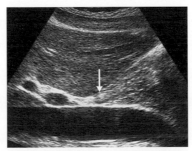

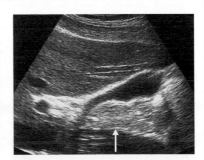

a Scan through the liver (L) and antrum (↓).

b The transducer was moved a little to the right, giving a section of the duodenal bulb (↓).

c The transducer was moved farther to the right. You now see a section of the second part of the duodenum (↑).

Defining the antrum and duodenum in transverse sections

The typical target appearance of the antrum is best displayed in longitudinal section at the inferior border of the liver. Locate this view, then rotate the transducer under vision to a transverse scan (Fig. 8.**22**).

*Fig. 8.**22*** ***Defining the antrum in transverse section***

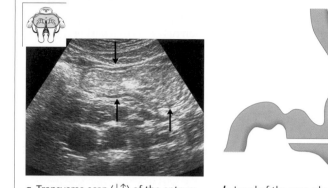
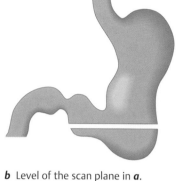

a Transverse scan (↓↑) of the antrum.   *b* Level of the scan plane in *a*.

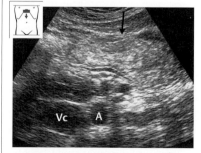

Fig. 8.**23**   **Course of the antrum, duodenal bulb, and second part of the duodenum.** The arrow indicates the scan plane in Fig. 8.**22**. The slices in the right part of the figure show the low-projecting antrum (A). The slices on the left depict the duodenal bulb (B), which initially runs cephalad, followed by the second part of the duodenum (D), which curves downward.

Note the position of the section. It passes through the lower part of the antrum, i.e., the inferior pole of the antrum lies in front of the image plane, while the pyloric opening into the duodenum is at a higher level and therefore is behind the image plane. The slices in Figure 8.**23** show the course of the antrum and the proximal segments of the duodenum.

Define the antrum in an upper abdominal transverse scan as shown in Fig. 8.**22 a**. Move the transducer lower, and follow the section of the antrum until it disappears (Fig. 8.**24**).

*Fig. 8.**24*** ***Scanning down the antrum in transverse sections***

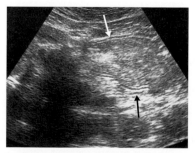
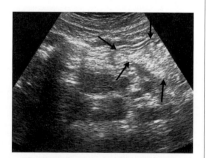

a Transverse scan of the antrum (↓).
A = aorta, Vc = vena cava.

b The transducer was moved to a slightly lower level. Antrum (↓↑).

c The transducer was moved lower. Chyme within the antrum (↓↑) creates a nonhomogeneous echo pattern.

Now return to the plane across the lower antrum (Fig. 8.**25 b**). Move the transducer higher and slightly to the right to demonstrate the pyloric region (Fig. 8.**25 c**). From there, trace the course of the duodenum by moving the transducer caudally in small increments (Fig. 8.**25 d**). Figure 8.**25 a** shows the progression of the scans.

Fig. 8.25 Defining the antrum, duodenal bulb, and second part of the duodenum in transverse sections

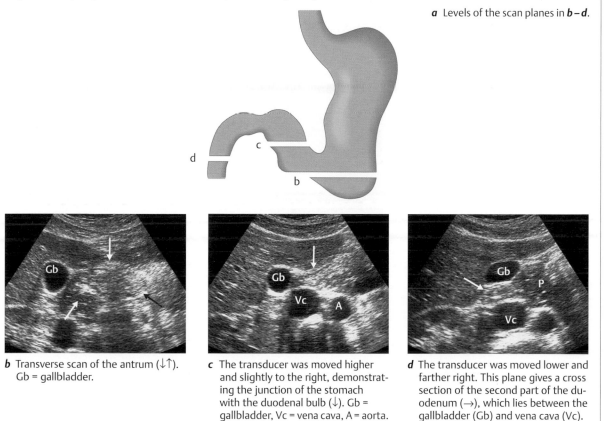

a Levels of the scan planes in **b**–**d**.

b Transverse scan of the antrum (↓↑). Gb = gallbladder.

c The transducer was moved higher and slightly to the right, demonstrating the junction of the stomach with the duodenal bulb (↓). Gb = gallbladder, Vc = vena cava, A = aorta.

d The transducer was moved lower and farther right. This plane gives a cross section of the second part of the duodenum (→), which lies between the gallbladder (Gb) and vena cava (Vc). P = pancreas.

Diaphragm

The left crus of the diaphragm descends along the left side of the aorta. The right crus descends to the right of the aorta and posterior to the vena cava (Fig. 8.**26**). Both crura can be identified as hypoechoic structures in transverse and longitudinal scans.

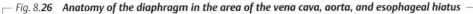

Fig. 8.26   Anatomy of the diaphragm in the area of the vena cava, aorta, and esophageal hiatus

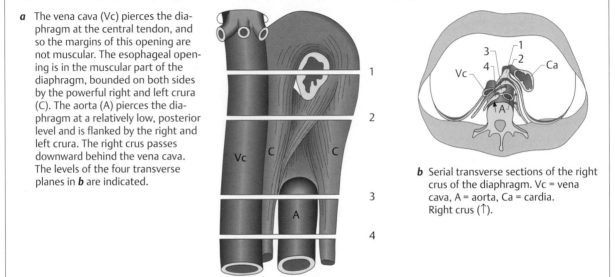

a The vena cava (Vc) pierces the diaphragm at the central tendon, and so the margins of this opening are not muscular. The esophageal opening is in the muscular part of the diaphragm, bounded on both sides by the powerful right and left crura (C). The aorta (A) pierces the diaphragm at a relatively low, posterior level and is flanked by the right and left crura. The right crus passes downward behind the vena cava. The levels of the four transverse planes in **b** are indicated.

b Serial transverse sections of the right crus of the diaphragm. Vc = vena cava, A = aorta, Ca = cardia. Right crus (↑).

Imaging the diaphragm in transverse sections

Place the probe transversely on the epigastrium and display a cross section of the aorta. Angle the scan steeply upward until you find the point where the aorta enters the chest cavity behind the heart. Then move the scan slowly down the aorta. Locate the entry of the esophagus into the abdominal cavity. Identify the hypoechoic band of the diaphragm between the gastroesophageal junction and the aorta. This band extends posteriorly on the right side (Fig. 8.**27 a, b**).

Now move the transducer lower while watching the diaphragm. Identify the right crus and left crus, which descend either side of the aorta. The right crus passes behind the vena cava (Fig. 8.**27 c**).

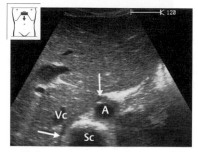

Fig. 8.27 **Defining the diaphragm in transverse sections**

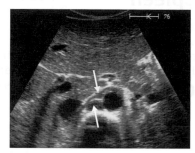

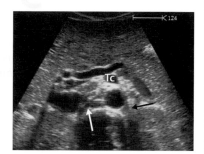

a High transverse scan. The powerful muscles of the diaphragm ($\downarrow\rightarrow$) are seen anterior to the aorta and posterior to the vena cava. A = aorta, Vc = vena cava, Sc = spinal column.

b The transducer was moved to a slightly lower level. You see the right crus of the diaphragm ($\uparrow$), which runs laterally behind the vena cava. An enlarged lymph node ($\downarrow$) is also seen.

c The transducer was moved lower. The crura ($\uparrow\leftarrow$) can be identified on both sides of the aorta and posterior to the vena cava. Tc = celiac trunk.

Imaging the diaphragm in longitudinal sections

Define the aorta in longitudinal section. Just anterior to the aorta, between that vessel and the gastroesophageal junction, you can clearly identify the powerful, hypoechoic musculature of the diaphragm, which extends relatively far inferiorly, almost to the level of the celiac trunk (Fig. 8.**28 a**). Move the transducer to the right, defining the vena cava in longitudinal section. Identify the right crus of the diaphragm posterior to the vena cava (Fig. 8.**28 b**).

Fig. 8.28 **Defining the diaphragm in longitudinal sections**

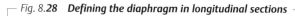

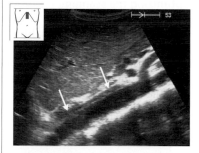

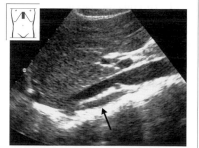

a Longitudinal scan over the aorta. The diaphragm ($\downarrow\downarrow$) is clearly visible anterior to the aorta.

b Longitudinal scan over the vena cava. The diaphragm ($\uparrow$) is clearly seen posterior to the vena cava.

Defining the spleen in longitudinal sections

Image the spleen in longitudinal section, and angle the transducer in an effort to obtain the best possible view. Now angle the scan posteriorly and see how the section of the spleen becomes smaller (Fig. 9.**4 b**). Angle the transducer back toward the front, and watch the hilar vessels come into view (Fig. 9.**4 c**). Continue scanning anteriorly until the section of the spleen becomes smaller again (Fig. 9.**4 d**) and finally disappears.

Defining the spleen in transverse sections

Image the spleen in the familiar longitudinal section and rotate the transducer under vision to a transverse scan (Fig. 9.**5 a**). Scan upward by angling the transducer cephalad, and then scan all the way down through the spleen in transverse sections (Fig. 9.**5 b – d**).

Fig. 9.5   Transverse flank scans of the spleen

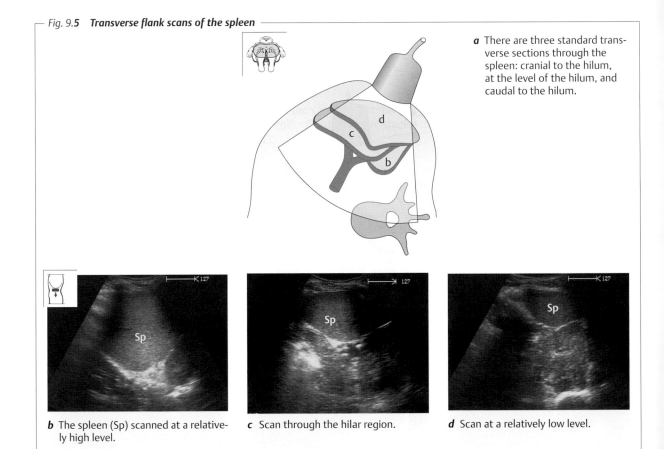

a There are three standard transverse sections through the spleen: cranial to the hilum, at the level of the hilum, and caudal to the hilum.

b The spleen (Sp) scanned at a relatively high level.

c Scan through the hilar region.

d Scan at a relatively low level.

Organ Details

LEARNING GOALS

➤ Evaluate the shape of the spleen.
➤ Determine the size of the spleen.
➤ Evaluate the echo pattern of the spleen.

Shape of the spleen

In shape, the spleen resembles a spherical segment whose convexity is related to the diaphragm superiorly, posteriorly, and laterally. It has impressions for the kidney (posteromedially), stomach (anteromedially), and colon (inferiorly) (Fig. 9.**6**). The hilar vessels are located between the stomach and kidney (see Fig. 9.**26 a**). The spleen is somewhat variable in its shape, however; it may be elongated or plump and occasionally shows deep constrictions (Fig. 9.**7**).

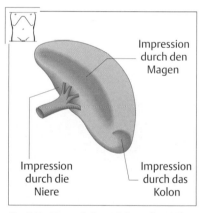

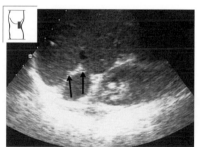

Fig. 9.7 **Constrictions of the spleen** (↑↑).

*Fig. 9.**6*** ***Frontal view of the spleen.*** The surface of the spleen bears impressions for the stomach, colon, and left kidney.

Determining the size of the spleen

For routine examinations, it is sufficient to measure the spleen in two dimensions. Define the spleen by scanning longitudinally from the flank as before. Angle the scan until it displays the splenic hilum. Measure the greatest longitudinal diameter in this view and the perpendicular diameter from the surface of the spleen to the hilum (Fig. 9.**8**).

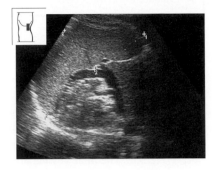

Fig. 9.**8** **Measuring the size of the spleen in a longitudinal flank scan.** The normal dimensions are 11–12 cm by 4 cm.

Enlarged spleen

Enlargement of the spleen is a feature of numerous disorders and is easily detected with ultrasound (Figs. 9.**9**, 9.**10**). The most frequent causes include portal hypertension, hematologic diseases, infectious diseases, amyloidosis, right-sided heart failure, and thrombosis of the splenic vein.

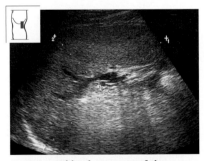

Fig. 9.**9** **Mild enlargement of the spleen in infectious mononucleosis.**

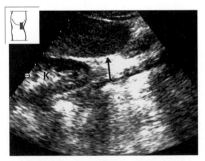

Fig. 9.**10** **Marked splenomegaly in spherocytosis.** The spleen (↑) extends past the lower pole of the kidney (K).

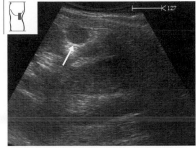

Accessory spleen

Accessory spleens are a common finding. Most are located close to the hilum (Fig. 9.**11**), and some are found at the lower pole (Fig. 9.**12**). Generally they are spherical and have the same echogenicity as the spleen.

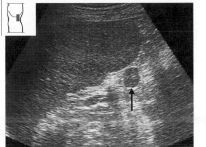

*Fig. 9.**11*** ***Accessory spleen (↑) close to the hilum.***

*Fig. 9.**12*** ***Accessory spleen (↑) at the lower pole.***

Echo pattern

KEY POINT

The normal spleen is slightly less echogenic than the liver.

The normal spleen has a homogeneous texture that is slightly less reflective than the liver. Vessels can be identified only in close proximity to the hilum.

Table 9.**1**   Differential diagnosis of diffuse splenic changes

Diffuse changes in the spleen

Lymphoma can cause a diffuse, fine, or coarsely nodular nonhomogeneity of the splenic echo pattern (Figs. 9.**13** – 9.**15**). In patients with splenomegaly due to portal hypertension, a homogeneous increase in echogenicity is often seen. Table 9.**1** lists the diagnoses that should be considered when diffuse splenic changes are found.

Infectious diseases

Connective tissue diseases

Hematologic diseases

Portal hypertension

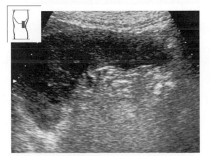

*Fig. 9.**13*** ***Hodgkin's disease infiltrating the spleen.*** Nonhomogeneous echo pattern.

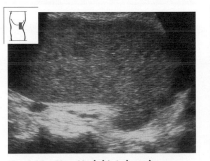

*Fig. 9.**14*** ***Non-Hodgkin's lymphoma infiltrating the spleen.*** The spleen exhibits a coarsely nodular, nonhomogeneous echo pattern.

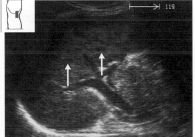

*Fig. 9.**15*** ***Non-Hodgkin's lymphoma in HIV infection.*** Numerous small, rounded, hypoechoic infiltrates (↑↑) are visible in the spleen.

Table 9.**2**   Circumscribed splenic changes

Calcification
Hemangioma
Metastases
Lymphoma
Infarction
Cyst
Abscess
Rupture/hematoma

Focal changes in the spleen

Circumscribed changes in the spleen are very rare. Often they cannot be diagnosed based on sonographic findings alone. The lesions that produce focal changes are listed in Table 9.**2**.

Calcifications. Calcifications in the spleen appear as hard, sharply circumscribed echoes that cast an acoustic shadow (Figs. 9.**16**, 9.**17**). They may occur as sequelae to infections (tuberculosis), hematomas, metastases, or hemangiomas.

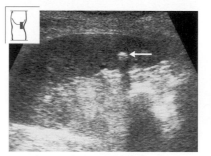

*Fig. 9.**16**   **Splenic calcification.*** Small, hard, spherical density with an acoustic shadow (←).

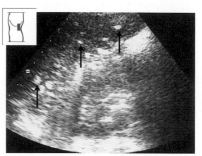

*Fig. 9.**17**   **Splenic calcification.*** Multiple stippled lesions of calcific density (↑↑↑) in a patient with a prior history of tuberculosis.

Echogenic lesions. Echogenic, non-shadowing splenic lesions may be hemangiomas (Fig. 9.**18**) or splenic metastases (Fig. 9.**19**).

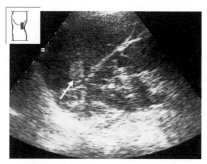

*Fig. 9.**18**   **Small hemangioma (↑).***

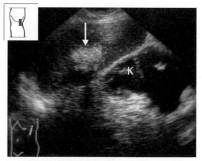

*Fig. 9.**19**   **Metastasis (↓).*** Severe hydronephrosis (K) is noted as an incidental finding.

Hypoechoic lesions. Hypoechoic lesions of homogeneous or nonhomogeneous texture are seen in association with metastases (Figs. 9.**20**, 9.**21**), infiltration of the spleen by lymphoma, and splenic infarction (Fig. 9.**22**).

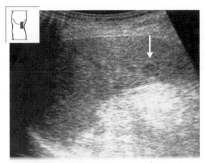

*Fig. 9.**20** Splenic metastasis (↓) from colon carcinoma.*

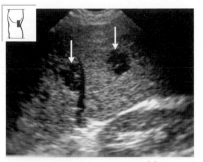

*Fig. 9.**21** Splenic metastases (↓↓) from a malignant melanoma.*

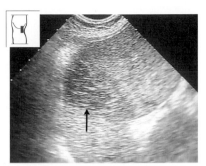

*Fig. 9.**22** Splenic infarction (↑).*

Echo-free lesions. Usually a splenic cyst is easily identified as a rounded, echo-free structure with well-defined margins (Fig. 9.**23**). Abscesses, on the other hand, appear as irregular, nonhomogeneous lesions that contain some internal echoes (Fig. 9.**24**).

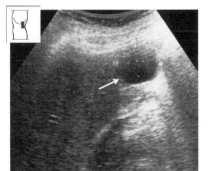

*Fig. 9.**23** Splenic cyst (↑).*

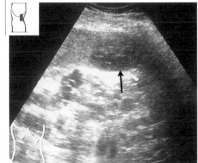

*Fig. 9.**24** Splenic abscess (↑).*

Anatomical Relationships

LEARNING GOAL

➤ Demonstrate the topography of the spleen in relation to the pleura, lung, colic flexure, stomach, kidney, and pancreas.

In locating the spleen, you have already become familiar with the adjacent gas-containing organs (Fig. 9.**25**). These structures are largely responsible for the difficulties in scanning the spleen. The left costodiaphragmatic recess extends beyond the upper pole of the spleen superiorly, laterally, and posteriorly. The colic flexure borders the lower pole of the spleen inferiorly and medially, and the stomach covers the spleen anteriorly and medially. The left kidney is posteroinferior to the spleen. The tail of the pancreas extends to the splenic hilum, or more accurately to a point anterior and inferior to the hilum. This allows the spleen to be used as an acoustic window for scanning the pancreatic tail (see p. 150).

KEY POINT

The gas-containing organs that surround the spleen make the organ difficult to scan.

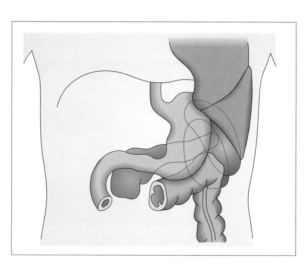

Fig. 9.25   Relationships of the spleen.

Relationship of the spleen to the pancreas, kidney, colic flexure, and stomach

The relation of the spleen to the pancreas was described earlier in the chapter on the pancreas (p. 150). Its relationship to the kidney, stomach, and left colic flexure are shown in Figure 9.**26**.

Fig. 9.26 Relationship of the spleen to the kidney, left colic flexure, and stomach

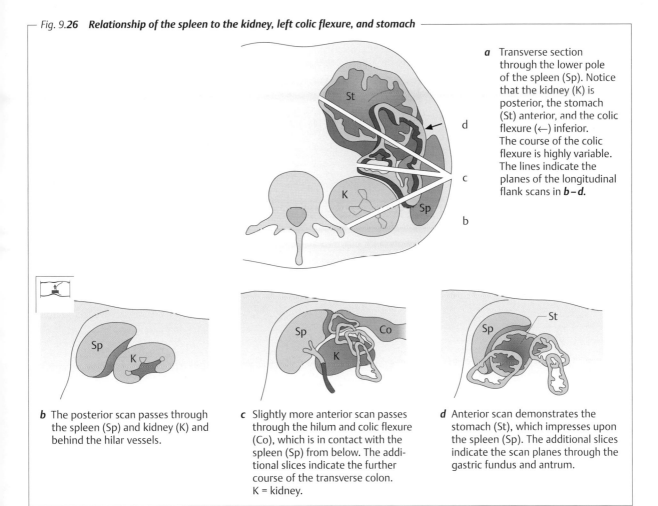

a Transverse section through the lower pole of the spleen (Sp). Notice that the kidney (K) is posterior, the stomach (St) anterior, and the colic flexure (←) inferior. The course of the colic flexure is highly variable. The lines indicate the planes of the longitudinal flank scans in *b–d.*

b The posterior scan passes through the spleen (Sp) and kidney (K) and behind the hilar vessels.

c Slightly more anterior scan passes through the hilum and colic flexure (Co), which is in contact with the spleen (Sp) from below. The additional slices indicate the further course of the transverse colon. K = kidney.

d Anterior scan demonstrates the stomach (St), which impresses upon the spleen (Sp). The additional slices indicate the scan planes through the gastric fundus and antrum.

Defining the relationships of the spleen to the kidney, colic flexure, and stomach in longitudinal sections

Start by imaging the spleen and left kidney in a longitudinal flank scan. Picture the location of the scan plane. It is relatively far posterior, behind the hilar vessels (Fig. 9.**27 a**). Angle the transducer a little anteriorly, bringing the hilar vessels into view. Look for the chaotic pattern of the colic flexure on the right (caudal) side of the image (Fig. 9.**27 b**). When you scan farther forward, in a plane anterior to the hilar vessels, the chaotic pattern of the stomach comes into view (Fig. 9.**27 c**).

Fig. 9.**27** *Defining the relations of the spleen to the kidney, colon, and stomach*

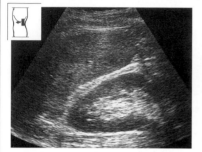 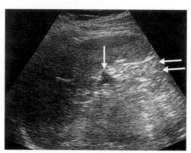 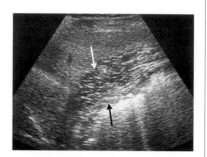

a Posterior scan of the spleen and kidney.

b Slightly more anterior scan demonstrates the splenic vein (↓) and colon (←←).

c Anterior scan of the spleen and stomach (↑↓).

Relationship of the spleen to the pleura

The costodiaphragmatic recess extends over the low posterolateral aspect of the spleen. It is a capillary space in expiration, but in inspiration it is expanded by the air-filled lung (Fig. 9.**28 a**). For this reason, it is often easier to demonstrate the spleen in expiration.

Defining the relationship of the spleen to the pleura

Position the transducer for a longitudinal flank scan, and demonstrate the spleen and kidney in one section (Fig. 9.**28 b**). Have the patient take a deep breath and exhale. Observe how the expanded lung makes the spleen difficult to see during inspiration (Fig. 9.**28 c**).

Fig. 9.28 *Defining the relationship of the spleen to the pleura*

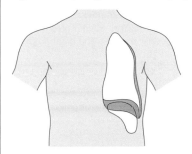 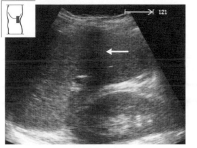 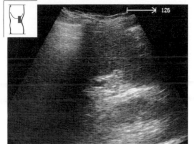

a The pleural space during expiration (white) and inspiration (gray). Notice that, during expiration, the pleural space is a narrow slit that is easy to scan through.

b The spleen during expiration. Rib shadow (←).

c Inspiration. The spleen is almost totally obscured by air.

Abnormalities associated with the spleen

Ascites and pleural effusion. Ascites appears as a fluid layer close to the splenic hilum (Fig. 9.**29**). With pleural effusion, the longitudinal flank scan demonstrates a fluid collection above the diaphragm (Fig. 9.**30**). This requires differentiation from ascites between the spleen and pleura (Fig. 9.**31**).

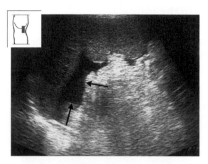

*Fig. 9.**29** **Ascites.** A fluid layer is seen along the visceral surface of the spleen in hepatic cirrhosis (↑←).

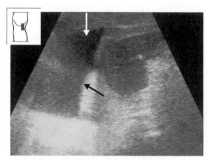

*Fig. 9.**30** **Pleural effusion (←↓).** A fluid collection is visible above the diaphragm.

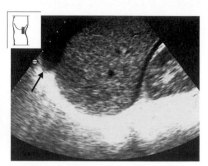

*Fig. 9.**31** **Ascites.** Fluid is also visible between the spleen and diaphragm (↑). Pancreatic carcinoma.

Portal hypertension (Figs. 9.**32**, 9.**33**). It is common to see collateral vessels at the splenic hilum in patients with portal hypertension.

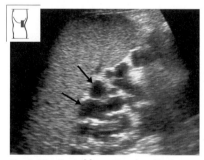

*Fig. 9.**32** **Portal hypertension.** Tortuous collateral vessels at the splenic hilum (↓↓).

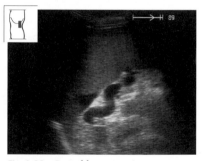

*Fig. 9.**33** **Portal hypertension.** The short gastric vein is greatly dilated (↑).

10 Kidneys

Organ Boundaries

LEARNING GOALS

➤ Locate and identify both kidneys.
➤ Demonstrate both kidneys in their entirety.

The kidneys are located in the retroperitoneum, one on each side of the spinal column. Ribs extend forward and downward over the kidneys, covering the upper third of each organ. The longitudinal axes of the kidneys converge toward the spinal column at an acute angle when viewed from behind and from the side (Fig. 10.**1 a, b**). Their transverse axes form an approximately 45 ° angle with the sagittal plane (Fig. 10.**1 c**).

Fig. 10.**1**   *The longitudinal and transverse axes of the kidneys*

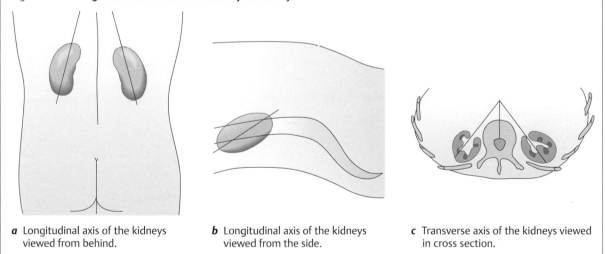

a Longitudinal axis of the kidneys viewed from behind.

b Longitudinal axis of the kidneys viewed from the side.

c Transverse axis of the kidneys viewed in cross section.

The liver, gallbladder, and pancreas are scanned primarily in transverse and longitudinal planes through the upper abdomen (Fig. 10.**2**).

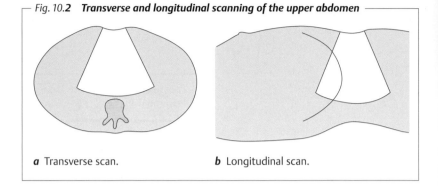

— Fig. 10.**2** **Transverse and longitudinal scanning of the upper abdomen** —

a Transverse scan.   *b* Longitudinal scan.

Renal scanning differs from this in several details because the kidneys are scanned from the flank. In the case of the right kidney, this means that a transverse scan is oriented as if the viewer were looking up into the sectioned torso from below (Fig. 10.**3a**). A longitudinal scan is like looking from posterior to anterior (Fig. 10.**3b**).

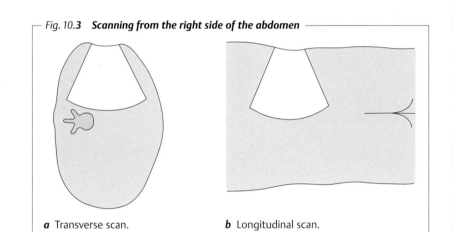

— Fig. 10.**3** **Scanning from the right side of the abdomen** —

a Transverse scan.   *b* Longitudinal scan.

In the case of the left kidney, a transverse scan is like looking up into the torso from below (Fig. 10.**4 a**), as on the right side. But a longitudinal scan from the left side is like looking from anterior to posterior (Fig. 10.**4 b**).

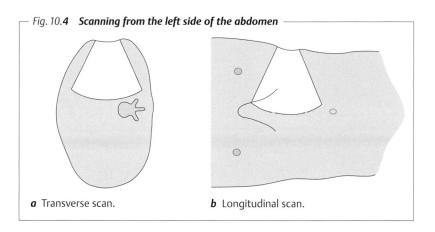

*Fig. 10.**4*** ***Scanning from the left side of the abdomen***

a Transverse scan.   *b* Longitudinal scan.

Locating the right kidney

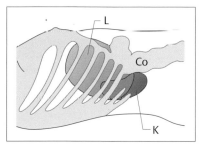

Fig. 10.**5** ***Lateral approach to the right kidney (K).*** The ribs and colon (Co) obstruct vision, while the liver (L) provides an acoustic window.

The right kidney lies posteriorly in an angle between the spinal column, musculature, and right lobe of the liver (Fig. 10.**5**). The right hepatic lobe extends laterally to the lower third of the kidney. The kidney is covered anteriorly by the right lobe, and its lower half in particular is covered by the right colic flexure and duodenum. Generally, then, the best approach is to scan the right kidney through the intercostal spaces from the posterolateral side and to use the liver as an acoustic window. Occasionally, however, you can obtain a clear view of the right kidney by scanning from the anterior side in thin, non-bloated patients.

Barriers to scanning

Visualization of the right kidney is obstructed by the 11th and 12th ribs and bowel gas.

Optimizing the scanning conditions

In most cases it is very helpful to have the subject take a deep breath. The kidney will move as much as several centimeters with respiratory excursions. Also, the left lateral decubitus position is preferred for renal scanning and may be supported by placing a roll beneath the contralateral side ("scoliosis" position). The ipsilateral arm can be raised to widen the intercostal spaces.

Organ identification

Place the transducer approximately on the posterior axillary line. Improve scanning conditions by using the maneuvers described above. Angle the scan slightly toward the head (Fig. 10.**6**). Define the kidney in an approximate longitudinal scan. Keep in mind that the image on the screen represents a posterior-to-anterior view of the body. Figure 10.**7** illustrates the typical appearance of this scan.

You should understand that this scan does not provide either an exact longitudinal or transverse view of the kidney, as it is slightly oblique. For the time being, however, it is entirely adequate for identifying the organ.

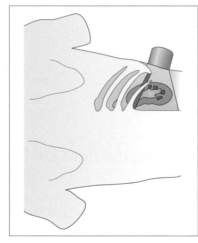

Fig. 10.**6** **Locating the right kidney.**

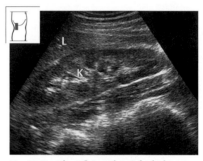

Fig. 10.**7** **Identifying the right kidney.** K = kidney, L = liver.

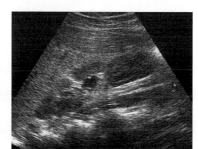
Imaging the entire right kidney

Longitudinal flank scan of the right kidney

Once you have defined the right kidney in an approximately longitudinal scan on the midaxillary line as described above, scan slowly across the organ from its posterior to anterior border, repeating this pass several times (Figs. 10.**8**, 10.**9**). Notice how the renal section becomes larger and then smaller as you scan through the organ. Notice, too, whether the scan covers the entire kidney; if it does not, examine the upper pole first and then scan the lower pole. Overlying ribs are not a serious problem, as you can examine the hidden portions of the kidney in a second pass.

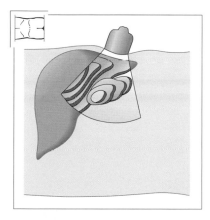

*Fig. 10.**8** Longitudinal flank scan: the beam is swept across the right kidney from posterior to anterior.*

*Fig. 10.**9** Longitudinal flank scan of the right kidney*

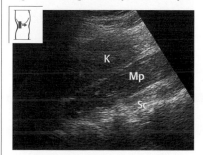

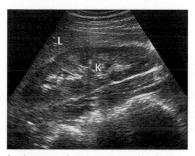

a Scan in a relatively posterior plane shows an indistinct section of the posterior right kidney.
K = kidney, Mp = psoas muscle, Sc = spinal column.

b The scan plane was moved a short distance anteriorly, displaying the kidney (K) in its maximum diameter.
L = liver.

c Scan in a more anterior plane. The renal section has become smaller again.

Transverse flank scan of the right kidney

Now rotate the transducer under vision to a transverse scan of the kidney (Fig. 10.**10**). Notice that the left side of the image is posterior and the right side is anterior. Place the transducer just below the costal arch or in a distal intercostal space. Sweep through the kidney from lower pole to upper pole, repeating this pass several times (Fig. 10.**11**). As you scan through the organ, make sure that you see a complete section of the kidney on the screen. Notice that the lower renal sections are closer to the transducer (i.e., the top of the image) than the higher renal sections because the long axis of the kidney is angled toward the spine.

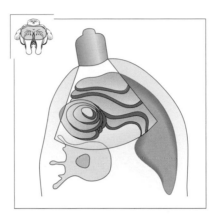

*Fig. 10.**10** Transverse flank scan: the beam is swept through the kidney from lower to upper pole.*

*Fig. 10.**11** Transverse flank scan of the right kidney*

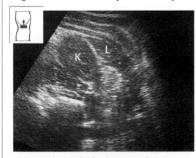

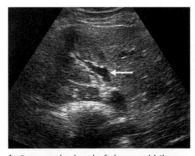

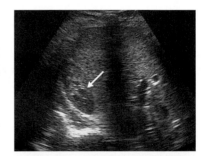

a Scan through the lower pole of the right kidney (K). L = liver.

b Scan at the level of the renal hilum (←). This scan displays the maximum renal diameter.

c Scan through the upper pole of the kidney (↑).

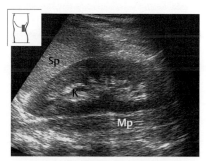

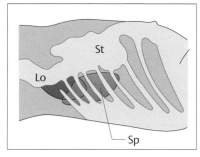

Fig. 10.12 Lateral approach to the left kidney. Colon (Co), stomach (St), and ribs obscure the left kidney, while the spleen (Sp) provides an acoustic window for scanning the upper pole.

Locating the left kidney

The left kidney lies posteriorly in an angle between the spinal column, musculature, and spleen (Fig. 10.12). The spleen extends laterally to about the middle of the left kidney. The lower half of the kidney is covered by the descending colon and left flexure. The left flexure passes around the anterior surface of the kidney and is in contact with it. The stomach overlies the front of the upper pole. Like the right kidney, then, the left kidney is best scanned through a posterolateral approach using the intercostal spaces and spleen as acoustic windows. The left kidney is considerably more difficult to scan than the right kidney, however, mainly because of intervening gas.

Barriers to scanning

The main barriers to scanning the left kidney are the 11th and 12th ribs and gas in the stomach and bowel.

Optimizing the scanning conditions

The measures are the same as for the right kidney.

Organ identification

The technique for identifying the left kidney is analogous to that used on the right side. The protocol is basically the same (Fig. 10.13). Please note that a longitudinal flank scan on the left side displays the body section as if it were viewed from the front. This is opposite to the back-to-front perspective that you saw in the right renal scan. Figure 10.14 illustrates the typical appearance of the scan.

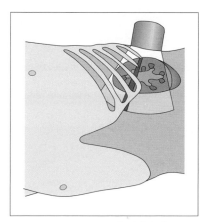

Fig. 10.13 Locating the left kidney.

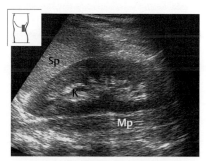

Fig. 10.14 Identifying the left kidney. K = kidney, Sp = spleen, Mp = psoas muscle.

Imaging the entire left kidney ──────

This technique is fully analogous to that used for imaging the right kidney.

Longitudinal flank scan of the left kidney

Figures 10.**15** and 10.**16** show how the kidney is scanned longitudinally from the flank. You scan completely through the kidney from back to front, repeating the pass several times.

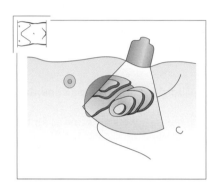

Fig. 10.15 Longitudinal flank scan: the beam is swept across the left kidney from posterior to anterior.

Fig. 10.16 Longitudinal flank scan of the left kidney

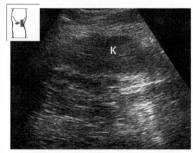

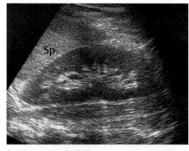

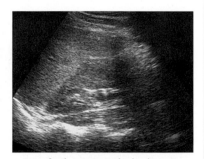

a Scan in a relatively posterior plane displays the posterior portions of the left kidney (K).

b Scan in a slightly more anterior plane passes through the maximum renal diameter. Sp = spleen.

c Scan farther anteriorly displays a smaller, anterior section of the kidney.

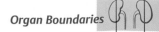

Transverse flank scan of the left kidney

The technique for scanning the left kidney in transverse sections is analogous to that used on the right side (Figs. 10.**17**, 10.**18**), but there is one essential difference; the left side of the screen image is anterior and the right side is posterior.

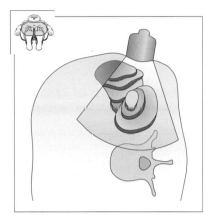

*Fig. 10.**17*** ***Transverse flank scan: the beam is swept through the left kidney from lower to upper pole.***

*Fig. 10.**18*** ***Transverse flank scan of the left kidney***

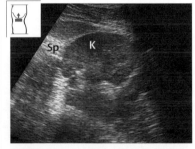

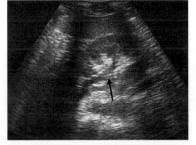

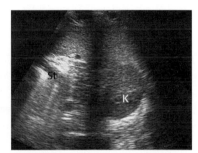

a Scan through the lower pole of the left kidney (K). Sp = spleen.

b Scan at the level of the renal hilum (↑).

c Scan through the upper pole of the kidney (K). St = stomach.

Abnormalities in locating the kidneys

Renal agenesis and ectopic kidneys. In renal agenesis, one kidney is absent while the contralateral kidney is usually enlarged. Ectopic kidneys may be found in the pelvis, but often they are obscured by intervening bowel gas.

Organ Details

➤ Evaluate the shape and size of the kidneys.
➤ Evaluate the renal parenchyma.
➤ Evaluate the renal sinus.

Size and shape of the kidneys

The kidney is a bean-shaped organ with a smooth surface that may have small indentations.

KEY POINTS

Renal dimensions have the following normal ranges:
Length 9 – 11 cm
Width 4 – 7 cm
Thickness 3 – 5 mm

Determining renal size with ultrasound

The kidney can be measured in three dimensions: length, width, and thickness. The longitudinal flank scan is best for determining renal length (Fig. 10.**19**), while the transverse flank scan is best for measuring width and thickness (Fig. 10.**20**). For convenience, however, both length and width are often measured in the longitudinal scan.

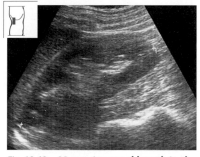

Fig. 10.*19* **Measuring renal length in the longitudinal flank scan.**

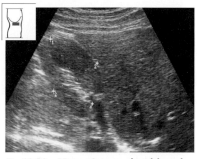

Fig. 10.*20* **Measuring renal width and thickness in the transverse flank scan.**

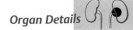

Changes in shape and size

Changes in shape. It is not uncommon to find surface indentations in the kidney, especially in older patients (Fig. 10.**21**). Pyelonephritis can also lead to surface indentations. The parenchyma of the left kidney often forms a bulge opposite the border of the spleen, creating a "dromedary hump" (Figs. 10.**22**, 10.**23**).

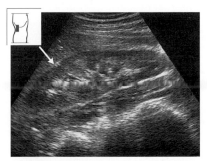

*Fig. 10.**21*** ***Normal finding.*** A small, echogenic indentation (↓) is seen between the upper and middle groups of calyces.

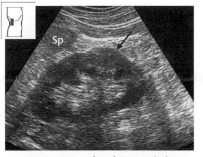

*Fig. 10.**22*** ***Dromedary hump.*** A bulge in the renal border (↓), isoechoic to the rest of the parenchyma, appears below the border of the spleen (Sp).

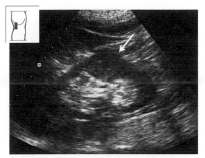

*Fig. 10.**23*** ***Dromedary hump.*** Renal parenchyma is relatively narrow and shows a slightly nonhomogeneous bulge (↓) opposite the lower border of the spleen.

In horseshoe kidney, the two kidneys are fused at their lower poles by an isthmus of parenchyma. This creates a "horseshoe" appearance when viewed from the front. The isthmus runs anterior to the aorta and may present as a mass when the aorta is scanned (see p. 42, Fig. 10.24). Hypernephroma can also produce a bulging renal contour (Figs. 10.25, 10.27). The differential diagnosis should include a parenchymal lobule, which is easily mistaken for a tumor (Fig. 10.26). Table 10.1 lists the sonographic features of hypernephroma.

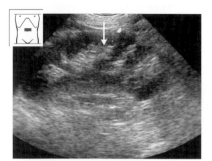

Fig. 10.24 **Horseshoe kidney.** The kidneys are fused by an isthmus of parenchyma (↓) that runs anterior to the aorta.

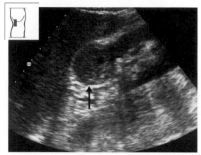

Fig. 10.25 **Hypernephroma.** The tumor appears as an approximately isoechoic, spherical mass (↑) bulging from the lower pole of the left kidney.

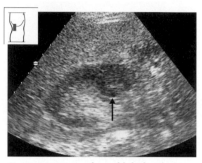

Fig. 10.26 **Parenchymal lobule.** The mass protruding into the renal pelvis is not a tumor but a lobule of renal parenchyma (↑), which appears rounded in this section.

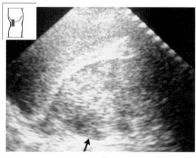

Fig. 10.27 **Hypernephroma.** Nonhomogeneous mass at the upper pole of the kidney.

Table 10.1 Sonographic features of hypernephroma

Hyperechoic and/or hypoechoic
Nonhomogeneous
Bulge in renal outline
Scalloped

Small kidney. The kidneys may become small or shrunken (Figs. 10.**28**, 10.**29**) as a result of chronic renal disease: glomerulonephritis, pyelonephritis, or renal artery stenosis. A small kidney can also result from ageing (Fig. 10.**30**) and occasionally occurs as a normal variant, in which case the contralateral kidney is usually hyperplastic.

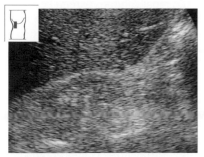

*Fig. 10.**28** **Shrunken kidney.*** Ultrasound shows a markedly small kidney with hyperechoic parenchyma and lack of corticomedullary differentiation.

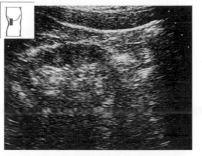

*Fig. 10.**29** **Shrunken kidney.*** In this case the renal architecture is intact.

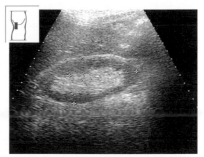

*Fig. 10.**30** **Age-related changes.*** The renal parenchyma becomes thinner with ageing, and there is an overall decrease in renal size.

Enlargement. Bilateral renal enlargement is seen in acute nephritis (Fig. 10.**31**) and renal shock as well as in chronic diseases such as diabetic nephropathy.

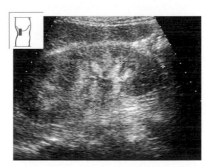

*Fig. 10.**31** **Mildly enlarged kidney in acute glomerulonephritis.***

Renal parenchyma and renal sinus

When you slice the kidney in half in the coronal plane, you first recognize the parenchyma and the renal sinus (Fig. 10.**32a**). The parenchyma consists of the cortex and medulla. The medulla is composed of 8 to 20 medullary pyramids (Fig. 10.**32b**). The cortex is 5–7 mm thick and forms the outer layer of the renal parenchyma. Fingers of cortex called the renal columns extend between the pyramids (Fig. 10.**32c**). The renal sinus contains the renal pelvis, a flattened sac into which the calyces open (Fig. 10.**32d**). The renal pelvis is surrounded by fat, connective tissue, and vessels (Fig. 10.**32e, f**).

Sonographic anatomy

We will now consider how the familiar anatomic structures of the kidney appear at ultrasound (Fig. 10.**32**). The anatomy is most clearly defined in a longitudinal flank scan that passes approximately through the center of the kidney.

*Fig. 10.**32** Sonographic anatomy of the kidney*

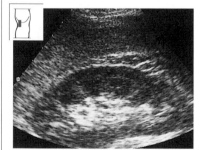

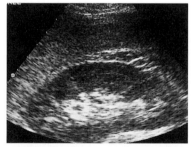

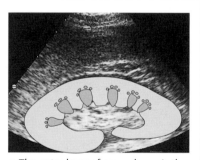

a Viewing a longitudinal scan of the kidney, you see the hypoechoic parenchyma surrounding the echogenic renal sinus, which is commonly referred to as the renal pelvis.

b On closer scrutiny, you can pick out the hypoechoic rounded triangles of the medullary pyramids. The tips of the pyramids project slightly into the renal pelvis.

c The outer layer of parenchyma is the cortex. Extensions from the cortex project between the pyramids as the renal columns.

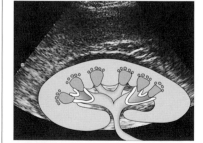

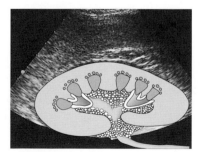

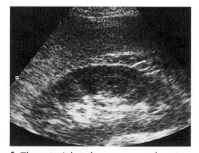

d The echogenic renal sinus consists of several anatomic structures. The first is the renal pelvis, which is usually collapsed but may be fluid-filled, appearing as an echo-free area.

e The renal pelvis is surrounded by copious fatty tissue.

f The arterial and venous vessels enter and exit the kidney at the hilum. The renal pelvis, fatty tissue, and vessels combine to form the echogenic image of the renal sinus.

Renal parenchyma

The renal parenchyma is relatively hypoechoic, appearing less echogenic than the liver and spleen. As you have already seen, you can distinguish the hypoechoic pyramids within the renal parenchyma.

Parenchymal width

The width of the renal parenchyma is subject to considerable variation. A normal range of 1.3 to 2.5 cm is reported (Fig. 10.**33**). The parenchymal diameter decreases with ageing, and the sinus broadens with increasing fat deposition. The sum of the anterior and posterior parenchymal diameters can be related to the width of the central echo complex and expressed as a ratio. A parenchymal–pelvic ratio of 1.6 : 1 is considered normal in young adults, and a 1 : 1 ratio is normal in older patients.

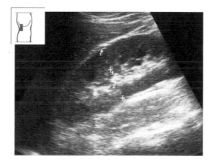

Fig. 10.**33** *Measuring the parenchymal width as the sum of the anterior and posterior widths.*

Now sweep the scan back and forth across the hepatorenal boundary several times (Fig. 10.**75**). As you do this, gain a spatial impression of how the organs are related to each other.

---

*Fig. 10.**75*** **Defining the relation of the kidney to the liver in the longitudinal flank scan**

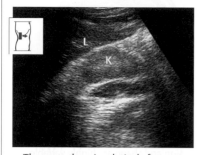 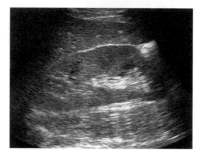 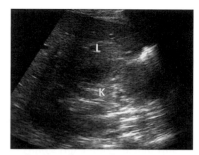

a The scan plane is relatively far posterior, demonstrating a small section of the kidney (K) and liver (L).

b The scan plane is at the center of the kidney.

c The scan plane is relatively far anterior, showing a large section of the liver (L) and a small section of the kidney (K).

It is easier to appreciate the hepatorenal boundary in patients with copious perirenal fat (Fig. 10.**76**) or if ascitic fluid has collected between the liver and kidney (Fig. 10.**77**).

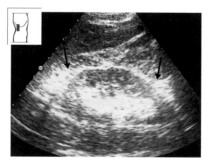 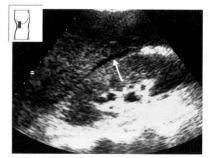

Fig. 10.**76**   *Copious perirenal fat (↓) in an obese subject.*

Fig. 10.**77**   *Ascites occupying the space between the kidney and liver (↑).*

Defining the relationship of the kidney to the liver in the transverse flank scan

Locate the kidney in a longitudinal flank scan. Rotate the transducer under vision to a transverse scan, and find a plane that shows the largest possible renal section plus a section of the liver. Take note of what you are seeing (Fig. 10.**78**) and picture how it would appear if the kidney were removed (Fig. 10.**79**).

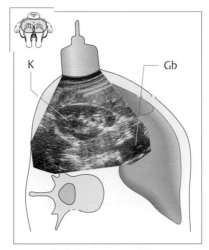

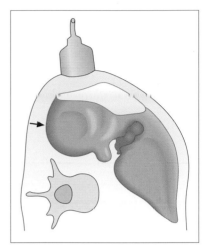

*Fig. 10.**78*** ***Transverse flank scan.*** The lateral border of the liver is close to the transducer. The posterior portions of the liver are displayed on the left side of the screen, the anterior portions on the right. The kidney (K) is posterior and medial to the liver. Gb = gallbladder.

*Fig. 10.**79*** ***Kidney has been removed to show the renal impression in the posterior inferior surface of the liver (→).***

Now scan up and down the hepatorenal boundary in transverse sections (Fig. 10.**80**). Gain a spatial impression of the boundary separating the organs.

*Fig. 10.**80*** ***Defining the relation of the kidney to the liver in the transverse flank scan***

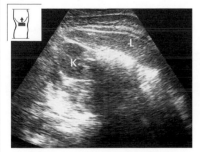

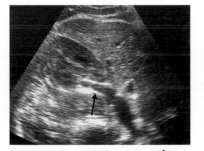

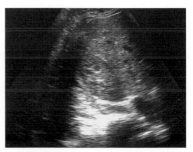

a Scan through the liver (L) and kidney (K) at the lower renal pole.

b Scan at the level of the hilum (↑).

c Scan through the upper pole of the kidney.

Relationship of the right kidney to the psoas and quadratus lumborum muscles

You have probably seen very little of these muscles since your anatomy class, and so a brief refresher may be needed. The psoas major muscle originates from the T12 through L4 vertebral bodies, runs forward and laterally over the ileum, and inserts on the greater trochanter of the femur. The quadratus lumborum muscle is a rectangular sheet that stretches between the 12th rib and the posterior iliac crest. Together, both muscles form the boundary of the posterior abdominal wall (Fig. 10.**81**).

Fig. 10.*81* *Location and course of the psoas muscle and quadratus lumborum*

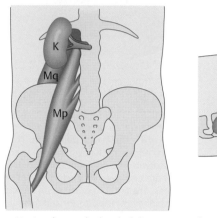

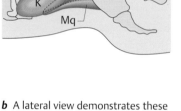

a Notice that at the level of the kidney (K), the psoas muscle (Mp) is medial to the kidney while the quadratus lumborum muscle (Mq) is posterior to the kidney.

b A lateral view demonstrates these relationships. K = kidney, Mp = psoas muscle, Mq = quadratus lumborum muscle.

Defining the relationship of the kidney to the quadratus lumborum and psoas muscles in the longitudinal flank scan

Because the quadratus lumborum muscle lies flat in the coronal plane, it usually cannot be identified with complete certainty. This is easier in the case of the psoas muscle. Scan longitudinally from the flank, and locate the renal section. Find a section that simultaneously displays the kidney and the echogenic band of the spinal column (Figs. 10.**82**, 10.**83**).

Fig. 10.82 *Longitudinal scan of psoas muscle between kidney and spinal column*

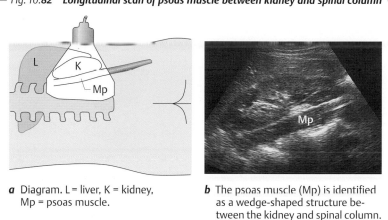

a Diagram. L = liver, K = kidney, Mp = psoas muscle.

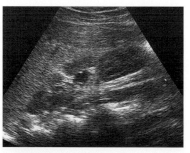

b The psoas muscle (Mp) is identified as a wedge-shaped structure between the kidney and spinal column.

Fig. 10.83 *Defining the relationship of the kidney to the quadratus lumborum and psoas muscles*

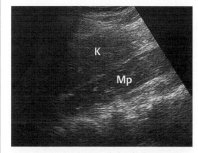

a Posterior section of the kidney (K) and psoas muscle (Mp).

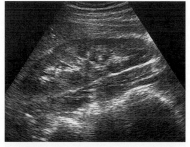

b Section through the middle of the kidney.

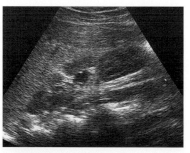

c Anterior section.

Defining the relationship of the kidney to the quadratus lumborum and psoas muscles in the transverse flank scan

While watching the monitor, rotate the transducer over the kidney to a transverse scan (Fig. 10.**84**). Sweep the scan up through the kidney and adjacent muscles (Fig. 10.**85**).

---

*Fig. 10.**84*** **Transverse scan of the psoas muscle between kidney and spinal column**

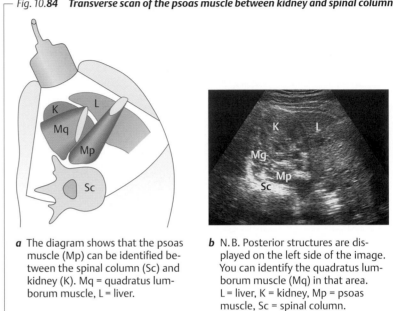

a The diagram shows that the psoas muscle (Mp) can be identified between the spinal column (Sc) and kidney (K). Mq = quadratus lumborum muscle, L = liver.

b N. B. Posterior structures are displayed on the left side of the image. You can identify the quadratus lumborum muscle (Mq) in that area. L = liver, K = kidney, Mp = psoas muscle, Sc = spinal column.

---

*Fig. 10.**85*** **Defining the relation of the kidney to the quadratus lumborum and psoas muscles in the transverse flank scan**

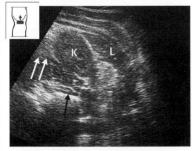

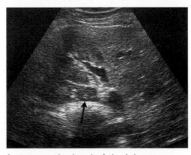

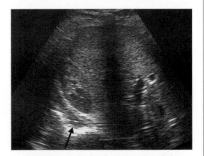

a Scan through the lower pole of the kidney. Both muscles are easily recognized. K = kidney, L = liver, psoas muscle (↑), quadratus lumborum muscle (↑↑).

b Scan at the level of the hilum. Psoas muscle (↑).

c Scan through the lower pole of the kidney. The section of the psoas muscle (↑) is still clearly visible.

Relationship of the right kidney to the colon ————

The right kidney is best visualized in lateral or posterior flank scans. It cannot always be seen from the anterior side due to overlying bowel gas. Please refer back to Figs. 10.**71 b** and 10.**72 b** and review the anatomy of the right colic flexure. The fact that the ability to demonstrate the kidney from the front varies in different individuals is due, in part, to the great variability of the colic flexure (Fig. 10.**86**).

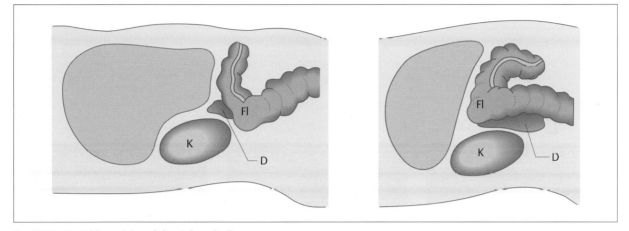

*Fig. 10.**86** Variable position of the right colic flexure.*
K = kidney, Fl = colic flexure, D = duodenum.

Defining the relationship of the kidney to the colon in the longitudinal flank scan

Position the transducer for a longitudinal flank scan and demonstrate the kidney (Fig. 10.**87 a, b**). Move the scan a little anteriorly, and watch the section of the kidney grow smaller. Meanwhile the colon appears anterior to the kidney at the inferior hepatic border (Fig. 10.**87 c, d**).

Fig. 10.87 **Defining the relation of the kidney to the colon in the longitudinal flank scan**

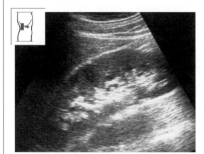
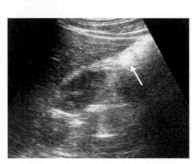
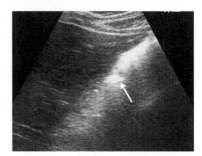

a The colic flexure (Fl) has been added to the diagram to show what is anterior to the image plane.

b Longitudinal flank scan of the kidney.

c The transducer was moved slightly anteriorly. The renal section becomes smaller, and a section of colon (↑) appears anterior to the kidney.

d The transducer was moved farther anteriorly. The air-filled colic flexure (↑) is visible at the inferior hepatic border.

Relationship of the right kidney to the gallbladder

You already learned about the relation of the right kidney to the gallbladder when you examined the gallbladder with intercostal flank scans (Fig. 6.**6**, p. 110). The relationship between the two organs can be difficult for the beginner to understand. Take another look at Fig. 10.**71**. The gallbladder lies anterior and slightly medial to the kidney. Figure 10.**88 a** shows the organs viewed from below, as in a transverse scan. Lateral views are shown in Fig. 10.**88 b – d**.

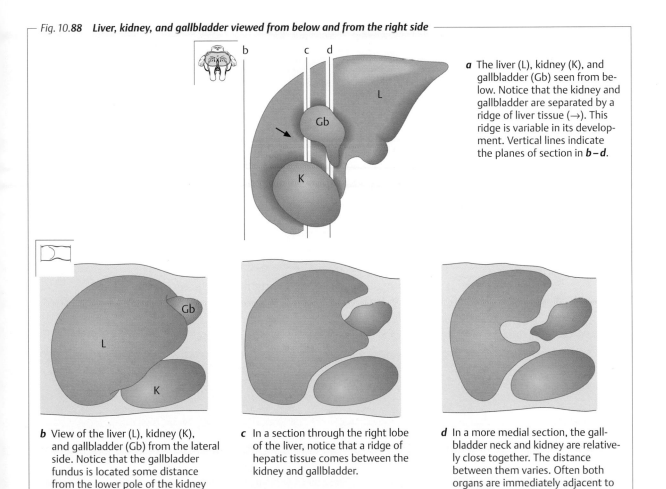

Fig. 10.**88** *Liver, kidney, and gallbladder viewed from below and from the right side*

a The liver (L), kidney (K), and gallbladder (Gb) seen from below. Notice that the kidney and gallbladder are separated by a ridge of liver tissue (→). This ridge is variable in its development. Vertical lines indicate the planes of section in *b – d*.

b View of the liver (L), kidney (K), and gallbladder (Gb) from the lateral side. Notice that the gallbladder fundus is located some distance from the lower pole of the kidney at this level.

c In a section through the right lobe of the liver, notice that a ridge of hepatic tissue comes between the kidney and gallbladder.

d In a more medial section, the gallbladder neck and kidney are relatively close together. The distance between them varies. Often both organs are immediately adjacent to each other.

Defining the relationship of the kidney to the gallbladder in the longitudinal flank scan

Locate the kidney in a longitudinal flank scan. This section is shown in Fig. 10.**89 a**. The posterior part of the liver and kidney were removed in Fig. 10.**89 b**. This drawing shows sections of the anterior portion of the liver and gallbladder viewed from behind.

Fig. 10.89   Sections through the liver, right kidney, and gallbladder

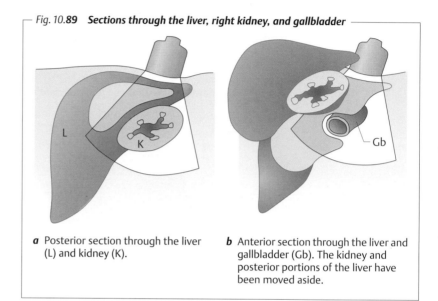

a Posterior section through the liver (L) and kidney (K).

b Anterior section through the liver and gallbladder (Gb). The kidney and posterior portions of the liver have been moved aside.

Perform this series of scans with the transducer (Fig. 10.**90**).

Fig. 10.90   Defining the relationship of the kidney to the gallbladder in the longitudinal flank scan

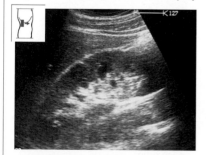 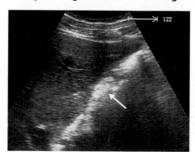 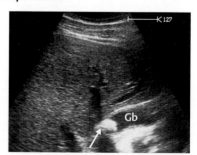

a Scan through the kidney.

b The scan was moved anteriorly past the kidney, demonstrating hepatic tissue with bowel gas (←) below it.

c The scan was moved farther anteriorly. The gallbladder (Gb) appears at the inferior border of the liver. The gallstone (↑) is an incidental finding.

Defining the relationship of the kidney to the gallbladder in the transverse flank scan

Demonstrate the liver and right kidney in a transverse flank scan (Fig. 10.**91 a**, **b**). Angle the scan upward and watch the gallbladder come into view (Fig. 10.**91 c, d**).

*Fig. 10.**91*** *Defining the relationship of the kidney to the gallbladder in the transverse flank scan*

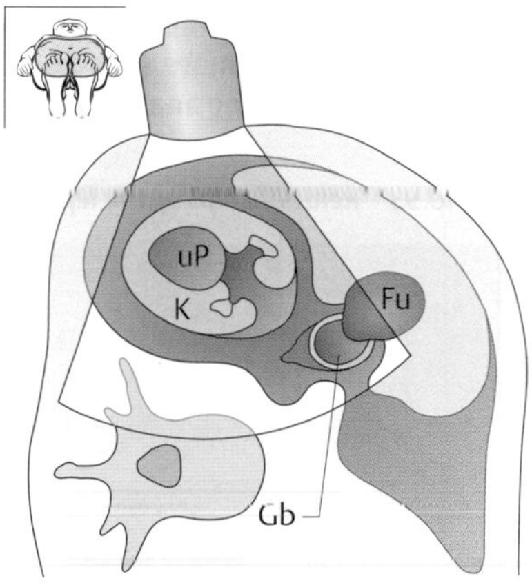

a Transverse section at the level of the renal hilum. Notice that the scan plane also cuts the gallbladder (Gb) anterior to the kidney (K). The upper renal pole and gallbladder neck are close together. The lower renal pole (uP) and gallbladder fundus (Fu) — both drawn in front of the image plane — are relatively far apart.

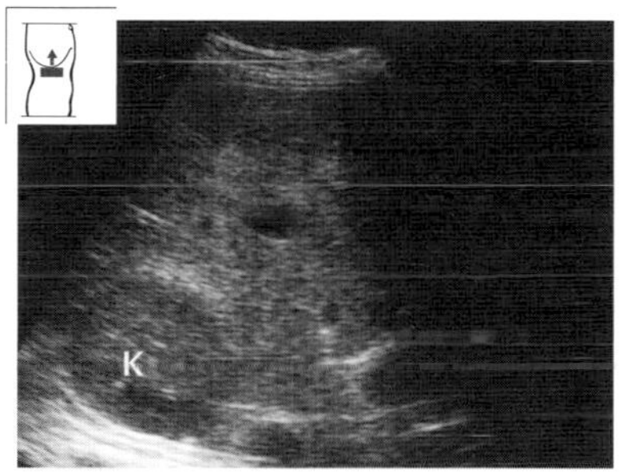

b Scan of the kidney at about the level of the renal hilum (K).

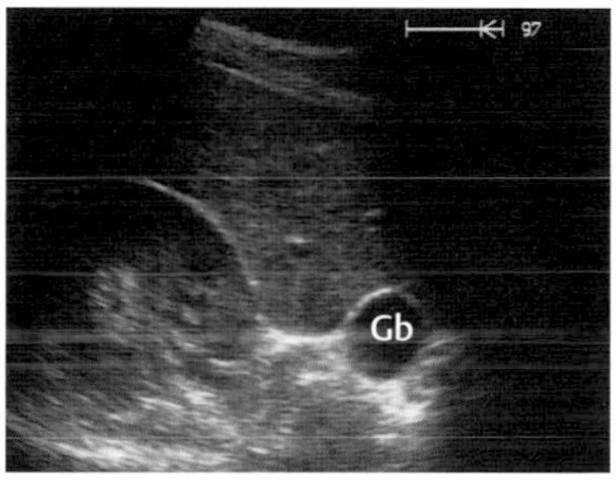

c Scan at a slightly higher level brings the gallbladder (Gb) into view.

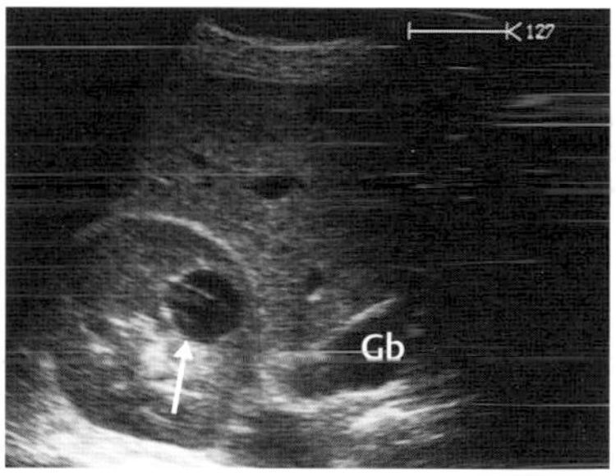

d Scan through the upper renal pole displays a relatively large section of the gallbladder (Gb). A renal cyst (↑) is noted as an incidental finding.

Epigastrium and pancreas

Examination of the epigastrium and pancreas proceeds in two steps:
1 Survey in longitudinal scans.
2 Survey in transverse scans.

Reporting guidelines

Large vessels and lymph node groups appear normal.
Marked aortic sclerosis is seen.
Atheromatous plaques are seen in the aorta, at the origin of the celiac trunk.
Aneurysmal dilatation of the aorta is noted below the renal arteries, ... cm in diameter, partially thrombosed, extension of aneurysm for ... cm.
Normal appearance of the vena cava.
➤ Vena cava shows normal caliber changes with respiration.
➤ Vena cava shows no caliber changes with respiration.

The splenic vein is:
➤ easily compressible,
➤ poorly compressible.

The pancreas is:
➤ clearly visualized,
➤ poorly visualized.

The head and body of the pancreas are well-defined, the tail is obscured by gas.
The pancreas cannot be adequately visualized due to bowel gas and obesity.
No large masses are seen.
Echogenicity is markedly increased, pancreatic lipomatosis.
The duct is not dilated.
The head of the pancreas contains several foci of calcific density, ... mm in size.
No masses are seen in the region of the pancreas.

Midabdomen

Examination of the midabdomen proceeds in two steps:
1 Survey in longitudinal scans.
2 Survey in transverse scans.

Lower abdomen

Examination of the lower abdomen proceeds in six steps:
1 Suprapubic longitudinal scans.
2 Suprapubic transverse scans.
3, 4 Longitudinal parailiac scans, right and left.
5, 6 Transverse parailiac scans, right and left.

Reporting guidelines

General examination of the lower abdomen is straightforward.
No evidence of free fluid.
Cul-de-sac appears normal.

EPIGASTRIUM AND PANCREAS

Aorta
– Diameter
– Wall
– Pulsations
– Vascular origins
  Celiac trunk
  Superior mesenteric artery

Lymph node groups
– Para-aortic
– Paracaval
– Celiac trunk

Vena cava
– Diameter
– Undulations
– Compressibility

Splenic vein
– Diameter
– Compressibility

Pancreas
– Shape
– Size
  Head
  Body
  Tail
– Pattern
– Pancreatic duct

MIDABDOMEN

Aorta
– Bifurcation

Vena cava
– Bifurcation

Lymph node groups

LOWER ABDOMEN

Bladder

Prostate

Uterus

Cul-de-sac

Iliac vessels

Description of Findings and Nomenclature

The outline below (Table 13.**1**) is intended to help the beginner in reporting ultrasound findings.

Table 13.**1** Description of findings and nomenclature

Criterion	Criterion
Size	Enlarged/reduced in size
	Thickened/thinned
	Expanded
	Dilated
	Shrunken
	Measurements in centimeters, taken in two or three dimensions
Shape	Plump
	Wavy
	Lobulated
	Scalloped
Borders	Sharp/indistinct
	Regular/irregular
	Smooth
Echo pattern	Hyperechoic/hypoechoic/echo-free
	Dense/rarefied
	Cystic
	Finely granular/coarsely granular
	Homogeneous/nonhomogeneous
Acoustic phenomena	Acoustic shadow
	Acoustic attenuation
	Acoustic enhancement
Accessibility to scanning	Good/poor/not seen
	Cannot be evaluated
	Completely/partially obscured by gas
	Cannot be found

Documentation

Every ultrasound examination should be documented with a written report and images.

Written report

The written report should cover both normal and abnormal findings, and any limitations should be stated. It should include a description of the findings, their interpretation, and a presumptive diagnosis. Sonographers should be hesitant in making a diagnosis, but there are lesions (e.g., cysts, gallstones) for which a definitive diagnosis can be offered. As a rule, referring physicians would rather have a conclusive report than a wordy, inconclusive account.

Example of a brief ultrasound report

Scanning conditions were good. The liver is normal in size and shape, with a sharp angle at the inferior border. Echogenicity is not increased. Hepatic veins are normal. No circumscribed masses. Gallbladder appears normal with no stones or wall thickening. Intra- and extrahepatic bile ducts appear normal. Both kidneys are normal for age in size and shape. No stones or obstruction. Spleen measures 4 × 11 cm and is not enlarged. Head and body of pancreas are well-defined, showing no abnormalities. Tail of pancreas cannot be clearly evaluated. Large vessels and lymph node groups appear normal. No free fluid.
  Summary: no abnormal findings.

Image documentation

KEY POINTS

Images are inherently worthless for documenting normal findings.

Images are excellent for documenting abnormal findings but must be supplemented by written notes or drawings to indicate location.

Several points should be noted with regard to the documentation of ultrasound images. First, it is important to understand why images are documented:
➤ to demonstrate a finding,
➤ to monitor the progression of disease,
➤ to document the examination for billing purposes.

Images are inherently worthless for documenting normal findings. Even a gallbladder with stones can be scanned in such a way that it appears to be clear. A normal-appearing image of the liver parenchyma does not exclude an adjacent metastasis.

  On the other hand, images are excellent for documenting abnormal findings (metastases, gallstones, etc.). However, all recorded images should be supplemented by written notes that describe the lesion and specify its location. The report should also include a drawing that indicates the scan plane.

Various media are available for the documentation of images:
➤ Printers
➤ Videotape
➤ Polaroid film
➤ 35-mm film
➤ Radiographic film
➤ Digital storage media

The medium of choice depends on the requirements of the situation and on the preferences and resources of the examiner.

Index